Dana-Farber Cancer Institute Handbook Series

Colorectal Cancer

Edited by

Jeffrey Meyerhardt
Assistant Professor of Medicine
Harvard Medical School
Medical Oncology Division
Dana-Farber Cancer Institute
Department of Medicine, Brigham and Women's Hospital
Boston, MA, USA

Mark Saunders
Consultant Oncologist
Clinical Oncology Department
Christie Hospital NHS Trust
Manchester, UK

Series Editor

Arthur T. Skarin
Associate Professor of Medicine
Harvard Medical School
Senior Attending Physician
Medical Director, Lowe Center for Thoracic Oncology
Dana-Farber Cancer Institute
Department of Medicine, Brigham and Women's Hospital
Boston, MA, USA

MOSBY

ELSEVIER

EDINBURGH LONDON NEW YORK OXFORD
PHILADELPHIA ST LOUIS SYDNEY TORONTO 2007

ELSEVIER
MOSBY

© 2003, Elsevier Limited.
© 2007 this compilation, Elsevier Limited. All rights reserved.
First published 2007

ISBN: 978 0 7234 3435 1

British Library Cataloguing in Publication Data
A catalogue record for this book is available from the British Library.

Library of Congress Cataloging in Publication Data
A catalog record for this book is available from the Library of Congress.

Note
Knowledge and best practice in this field are constantly changing. As new research and experience broaden our knowledge, changes in practice, treatment and drug therapy may become necessary or appropriate. Readers are advised to check the most current information provided (i) on procedures featured or (ii) by the manufacturer of each product to be administered, to verify the recommended dose or formula, the method and duration of administration, and contraindications. It is the responsibility of the practitioner, relying on their own experience and knowledge of the patient, to make diagnoses, to determine dosages and the best treatment for each individual patient, and to take all appropriate safety precautions. To the fullest extent of the law, neither the Publisher nor the Editors/Authors assume any liability for any injury and/or damage to persons or property arising out or related to any use of the material contained in this book.

The Publisher

Working together to grow
libraries in developing countries

www.elsevier.com | www.bookaid.org | www.sabre.org

ELSEVIER   BOOK AID   Sabre Foundation
             International

your source for books,
journals and multimedia
in the health sciences

www.elsevierhealth.com

The
Publisher's
policy is to use
paper manufactured
from sustainable forests

Printed in China

Contents

Preface

Colorectal cancer is the fourth most commonly diagnosed malignancy worldwide. Just over a million people are diagnosed every year, approximately half of whom will die from this cancer. The treatment of this illness has improved greatly over the past 20 years, leading to a steady decrease in overall mortality. This book carefully runs through both the basics of colorectal cancer and the advances we have made that have led to this improvement.

If we look back at the 1980s, the treatment options for colorectal cancer were very limited. Public awareness was poor and screening for this malignancy was virtually non-existent. Consequently, patients often presented late, and apart from surgery there was little we could do to really influence their outcome. The local recurrence rate for rectal cancer at this point was in the order of 40–50%. Various randomized trials were published in the next decade which showed that radiotherapy could reduce this figure to around 10%. Surgical techniques then improved with the advent of total mesorectal excision, and now a combination of this with a short course of preoperative radiotherapy can reduce the recurrence rate to less than 5%. For those clinicians who have witnessed the devastating effects of uncontrolled pelvic malignancy, this is a substantial and very welcome improvement.

With the advent of the new millennium, systemic therapies have improved. For approximately 40 years, all we had was 5-fluorouracil (5FU), which was given in all sorts of regimens. The median survival for patients with advanced disease was only 1 year at this point. The sequential use of irinotecan and oxaliplatin combined with 5FU raised this figure to more than 20 months. We now have even more options, including the epidermal growth factor receptor inhibitor cetuximab, and the vascular endothelial growth factor inhibitor bevacizumab. Patients can now regularly receive two lines and sometimes, if they are fit enough, even three of four different types of therapy. This has led to our breaking the 2-year median survival barrier for patients with advanced disease. This again is a substantial and very welcome improvement. More recently, trials have also shown that combination chemotherapy can improve a patient's outcome if it is used as an adjuvant.

Where do we go from here? Even with these advances over the past 20 years, colorectal cancer is still a devastating illness, and a 2-year median survival for patients with advanced disease is nothing to write home about. Improved pathological techniques and a more widespread use of screening will no doubt lead to the diagnosis of patients at an earlier stage. More efficacious and more convenient adjuvant therapies, which are targeted and better tolerated, will hopefully reduce the number of patients presenting with advanced disease. Cost may then be the main limiting factor.

Colorectal cancer is a disease of the western world. This obviously includes both the US and Europe. This book provides a real insight into the diagnosis, staging and treatment of patients with this illness that is very relevant to clinicians on both sides of the Atlantic.

Dr Mark Saunders
Consultant Oncologist
Clinical Oncology Department
Christie Hospital NHS Trust
Manchester, UK

Contributors

Joseph P. Eder, MD
Assistant Professor of Medicine, Harvard Medical School
Phase I Group
Medical Oncology Division
Dana-Farber Cancer Institute
Department of Medicine
Brigham and Women's Hospital
Boston, MA, USA

Matthew H. Kulke, MD
Assistant Professor of Medicine, Harvard Medical School
Medical Oncology Division
Dana-Farber Cancer Institute
Department of Medicine
Brigham and Women's Hospital
Boston, MA, USA

Janina A. Longtine, MD
Assistant Professor of Pathology, Harvard Medical School
Clinical Director, Molecular Biology Laboratory
Department of Pathology
Brigham and Women's Hospital
Boston, MA, USA

Jerrold R. Turner, MD, PhD
Associate Professor
Department of Pathology
The University of Chicago
Chicago, IL, USA

Tad Wieczorek, MD
Instructor in Pathology, Harvard Medical School
Department of Pathology
Brigham and Women's Hospital
Boston, MA, USA

Acknowledgements

The work of the associate editors of the *Atlas of Diagnostic Oncology* needs to be acknowledged. Dr Maxine Jochelson (currently Director of Oncologic Radiology and Women's Imaging, Cedars-Sinai Medical Center, Los Angeles, CA) and Dr Robert Penny (currently Director of Hematopathology, Community and St Vincent's Hospital of Indianapolis, IN) assisted with the first edition. Their immense help in organizing and evaluating the radiographic and pathology material for the chapters contributed significantly to the success of the *Atlas*. The work of the associate editors of the third edition, Dr Kitt Shaffer, currently of Cambridge City Hospital, Cambridge, MA and Dr Tad Wieczorek, Instructor in Pathology at Brigham and Women's Hospital, is also deeply appreciated. Their expertise was invaluable in emphasizing the illustrative and teaching aspects of the third edition. Without their hard work on the *Atlas of Diagnostic Oncology* this Handbook would not have been possible.

Acknowledgement also has to go to the editorial staff at Elsevier Ltd for their assistance in preparing the *Dana-Farber Cancer Institute Handbook Series*.

Introduction

Arthur T. Skarin

The likelihood of developing cancer during one's lifetime is one in two for males and one in three for females, based on the 1998–2000 Surveillance, Epidemiology and End Results (SEER) database.[1] The median age at cancer diagnosis is 68 years for men and 65 years for women. The overall 5-year relative survival rate for all patients is 62.7% with considerable variation by cancer site and stage at diagnosis. The variation in cancer statistics over recent years in the US is depicted in Figures 1.1 and 1.2. The American Cancer Society estimates that in 2006 the total number of new cases will be 1,399,790 with 564,830 deaths (see Figure 1.3).[2] The death rate from all cancers combined has decreased by 1.5% per year since 1993 among men and by 0.8% per year since 1992 for women. The mortality rate in men has also continued to decrease for the three most common sites (lung/bronchus, colorectal and prostate) as well as for breast and colorectal cancers in women. Death rates have decreased significantly for white, black and Asian/Pacific Islander males and females but not for American Indians, Alaska Nationals or Hispanics.[3] However, the decrease has been smaller among blacks compared with whites, resulting in an increased disparity between blacks and whites. Survival rates have been increasing for colorectal cancer in the past 40 years, undoubtedly related to improved screening and better treatments. Of interest, however, since 1999, cancer has surpassed heart disease as the leading cause of death for those under 85 years of age.[2] The reverse exists for those over age 85.

Worldwide, an estimated 11 million new cases and 7 million cancer deaths occurred in 2002, while nearly 25 million people were living with cancer.[4] Global disparities in cancer incidence, mortality and prevalence relate to genetic susceptibility and ageing, but also to modifiable risk factors such as tobacco abuse, infectious agents, certain dietary factors and physical activity. Other modifiable factors include overweight/obesity, urban air pollution, indoor smoke from household fires, unsafe sex, and contaminated injections in healthcare settings.[5] At least one-third of world cancer deaths are felt to be preventable. The associations of established causes of human cancers have been categorized as chemicals and

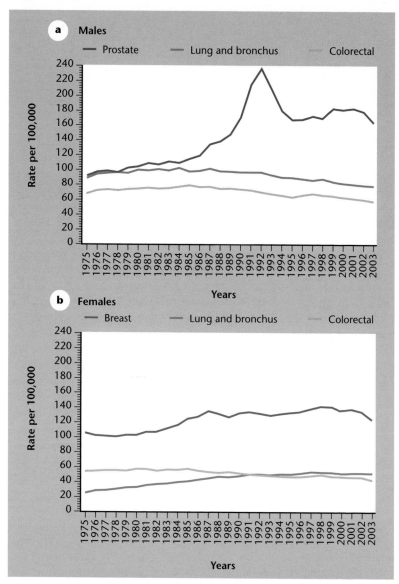

Fig. 1.1 Annual age-adjusted cancer incidence rates among (**a**) males and (**b**) females for selected cancers in the US, 1975 to 2003. Data from: Surveillance, Epidemiology, and End Results (SEER) program (http://seer.cancer.gov') SEER*Stat Database: Incidence – SEER 9 Regs Public-Use, Nov 2005 Sub (1973-2003), National Cancer Institute, DCCPS, Surveillance Research Program, Cancer Statistics Branch, released April 2006, based on the November 2005 submission.

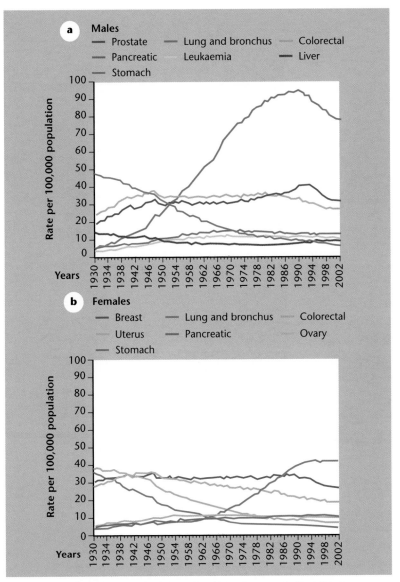

Fig. 1.2 Age-adjusted cancer death rates for selected cancers in the US between 1930 and 2002 for (**a**) males and (**b**) females. Source: US Mortality Public Use Data Tapes, 1960 to 2002, US Mortality Volumes, 1930 to 1959, National Center for Health Statistics, Centers for Disease Control and Prevention, 2005. Reproduced with permission from American Cancer Society. Cancer Facts and Figures 2006. Atlanta: American Cancer Society, Inc.

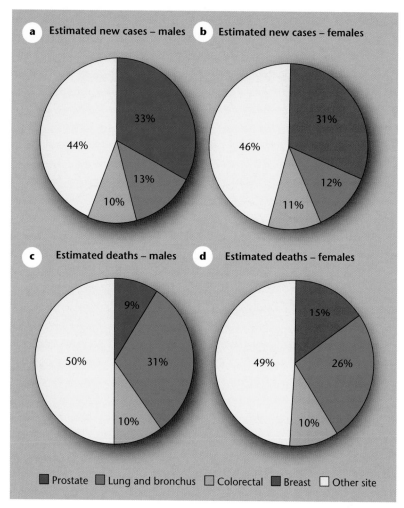

Fig. 1.3 Leading sites of new cancer cases and deaths – 2006 estimates. (**a**) Estimated new cases – males. (**b**) Estimated new cases – females. (**c**) Estimated deaths – males. (**d**) Estimated deaths – females. Source: American Cancer Society, Inc., Surveillance Research. Estimates of new cases are based on incidence rates from 1979 to 2002, National Cancer Institute's Surveillance, Epidemiology, and End Results program, nine oldest registries. Estimates of deaths are based on data from US Mortality Public Use Data Tapes, 1969 to 2003, National Center for Health Statistics, Centers for Disease Control and Prevention, 2006.

naturally occurring compounds, medicines and hormones, infectious agents and mixtures.[6] Since about 90% of all colorectal cancer cases and deaths are considered to be preventable, the aetiological factors are mainly modifiable risk factors.[7]

Because of the improvements in healthcare and other factors, there is an increasing ageing population in the US and many other countries in the world. It has been estimated that the proportion of people over age 65 years will increase from 12.6% in 2000 to 14.7% in 2015 and 20% in 2030 in the US.[8] This compares with 18.1% in Italy (used as a comparison as the oldest country in the world) in 2000, 22.2% in 2015 and 28.1% in 2030. Since the incidence of cancer increases with age, a rising number of cancer cases and deaths is predicted. Screening for cancer is therefore extremely important for early detection and subsequent cure. The annual screening recommendations by the American Cancer Society have been published.[9] Recommended screening studies for colorectal cancer include faecal occult blood testing (FOBT), flexible sigmoidoscopy, flexible sigmoidoscopy with FOBT, colonoscopy or double-contrast barium enema. Conventional colonoscopy remains more sensitive than other tests with a sensitivity for colorectal cancers >95%. Screening is recommended at age 50 for average-risk individuals and at an earlier age for those at higher risk because of family history of colorectal cancer or other factors.[10] About 6% of colorectal cancers are caused by recognizable hereditary germline mutations. The most frequent mutation involves the *APC* gene. Adenomas usually develop in the mid-teenage years of these patients with familial adenomatous polyposis (FAP);[11] colorectal cancer eventually occurs in virtually all patients. Screening at an early age with appropriate management is crucial to prevent subsequent colorectal cancer.

Cancer prevention is extremely important and the progress in information technology has been recently reviewed.[12] Chemoprevention studies have been carried out for several cancers and also recently reviewed.[13,14] Goals include integration of specific molecular biomarker expressions into the development of new agents for chemoprevention of early intraepithelial neoplasia. The molecular targets summarized in this AACR Task Force Report include anti-inflammatory/antioxidant agents, epigenetic modulation areas, and signal transduction modulation targets.[15] Six characteristics of neoplasms and the associated molecular targets that may be adversely affected by chemoprevention or definitive treatment programmes are noted in Table 1.1.[16] Chemoprevention of colorectal cancer, particularly with use of non-steroidal anti-inflammatory drugs (NSAIDs), is an area of intense research. In the US, celecoxib is

Table 1.1 Molecular biomarkers associated with neoplasia characteristics[16]

Evading apoptosis

BCL-2, BAX, caspases, FAS, TNF receptor, DR5, IGF/PI3K/AKT, mTOR, p53, PTEN, *ras*, IL-3, NF-κB

Insensitivity to antigrowth signals

SMADs, pRb, cyclin-dependent kinases, MYC

Limitless replicative potential

hTERT, pRb, p53

Self-sufficiency in cell growth

Epidermal growth factor, platelet-derived growth factor, MAPK, PI3K

Sustained angiogenesis

VEGF, basic fibroblast growth factor, $\alpha_v\beta_3$, thrombospondin-1, hypoxia-inducible factor-1α

Tissue invasion and metastasis

Matrix metalloproteinases, MAPK, E-cadherin

BAX, BCL-2 associated X protein
BCL-2, B cell lymphoma 2
DR5, death receptor 5
FAS, fatty acid synthase
hTERT, human telomerase reverse transcriptase
IGF, insulin-like growth factor
IL, interleukin
MAPK, mitogen-activated protein kinase
mTOR, mammalian target of rapamycin
NF, nuclear factor
PI3K, phosphatidylinositol 3-kinase
pRb, retinoblastoma protein
PTEN, phosphatase and tensin homologue deleted on chromosome 10
TNF, tumour necrosis factor
VEGF, vascular endothelial growth factor

approved by the US Food and Drug Administration to reduce the number of adenomatous colorectal polyps in FAP as an adjunct to usual care (e.g. endoscopic surveillance and surgery).[11]

With completion of the Human Genome Project new knowledge has become available about genetic variations that can help us to understand the family history as a risk factor for most cancer types. Identification of mutations in genes may identify individuals at high risk for certain cancers (*BRCA 1* & *2*, *P53*, *PTEN*, etc), and allow for early detection, as well as an understanding of the aetiological subtypes of cancer and inherited alterations in drug metabolism. This exciting field of molecular epidemiology may thus impact favourably on cancer prognosis.[17] The importance of the above underscores the need for collection and storage of adequate tissue for study.

The new information explosion in molecular biology has led to important discoveries in unique patterns of gene expression characteristic of certain malignancies.[18] This genetic expression profiling will be important not only for accurate diagnosis but for determining prognosis and candidates for certain therapies.[19]

Another new blossoming area of research is cancer proteomics.[20] As the result of carcinogenesis, abnormalities in protein networks extend outside the cancer cell to the tissue microenvironment in which exchange of cytokines, enzymes and other proteins occurs to the advantage of the malignant cell. These molecules can be identified and become the target for new diagnostic and/or therapeutic targets. Major progress is occurring in the proteomics field in discovery of biomarkers that may be useful in prediction of clinical response to anticancer therapy.[21]

Major research advances have not only occurred during the past few years in cancer biology, genetics prevention and screening, but also in cancer treatment. New standards of care for breast, lung, colorectal and other cancers became established during 2005.[22] There is also evidence of an increasing number of newer targeted therapies that can improve survival in some of the most common cancers but are also active against several other malignancies. This applies to adjuvant chemotherapy after surgery as well as advanced disease (see new and updated results in Chapter 4). Targeted therapy has advantages of oral administration for many agents and directed attack on cancer cells, sparing most healthy cells including the hair and bone marrow. For example, in advanced colorectal cancer, adding bevacizumab to the FOLFOX regimen appears to improve the prognosis. The new regimen was used in patients who had received previous chemotherapy and survival was increased by 17%.[23] Of note, a detailed review of new and future therapeutic targets has been recently published.[24] Also, multidisciplinary treatment guidelines from the National Comprehensive Cancer Network for colorectal cancer have been updated.[25]

The Dana-Farber Cancer Institute Atlas of Diagnostic Oncology was originally published in 1991 as a comprehensive reference and teaching aid in the various clinical, laboratory, pathological and radiological features of specific cancers. Because of the dramatic progress in understanding the molecular biology of cancer and the recent development of multiple chemotherapeutic agents. It became apparent that there was a need for a combination of the teaching aspects of the Atlas with a review and recommendations of modern therapeutic programmes available to cancer patients. Thus arose the new Dana-Farber Cancer Institute Handbooks of four common cancers – breast, colorectal, lung and prostate. Relevant sections of the 3rd edition of the Atlas have been updated and are now combined with a new chapter, which includes treatment strategies for the four major cancers listed above.

In each of our Handbooks, the authors will review important aspects of each cancer, including epidemiology, diagnostic work-up and staging evaluation, with photographic examples of pathology subtypes and clinical presentations, followed by an up-to-date detailed discussion of multimodality treatment programmes with current recommendations where necessary. In this book on colorectal cancer, Dr. Jeffrey Meyerhardt, attending physician on the Gastrointestinal Oncology Service at DFCI, will review various aspects of comprehensive treatment including the use of new drugs such as the targeted agents bevacizumab, cetuximab and panitumumab. The importance of patient symptom management and quality of life efforts will also be addressed.

REFERENCES

1. Gloeckler LA, Reichman ME, Riedel Lewis D, et al: Cancer survival and incidence from the Surveillance, Epidemiology, and End Results (SEER) program. Oncologist 2003; 8: 541–552.
2. Jemal A, Siegel R, Ward E, et al: Cancer statistics, 2006. CA Cancer J Clin 2006; 56: 106–130.
3. Jackson-Thompson J, Ahmed F, German RR, et al: Descriptive epidemiology of colorectal cancer in the United States, 1988–2001. Cancer 2006; 107 (5 Suppl): 1103–1111.
4. Kamangar F, Dores GM, Anderson WF: Patterns of cancer incidence, mortality, and prevalence across five continents: defining priorities to reduce cancer disparities in different geographic regions of the world. J Clin Oncol 2006; 24(14): 2137–2150.
5. Ezzati M, Henley SJ, Lopez AD, Thun MJ: Role of smoking in global and regional cancer epidemiology: current patterns and data needs. Int J Cancer 2005; 116: 963–971.
6. Neugent AI: Cancer epidemiology and prevention. Sci Am 2004; 12: 2–11.
7. Reed E, Ahmed F, Jackson-Thompson J, et al: Foreword: promoting the use of registry-based national cancer surveillance data for colorectal cancer prevention and control. Cancer 2006; 107 (5 Suppl): 1101–1102.
8. Yancik R: Population aging and cancer: a cross-national concern. Cancer J 2005; 11: 437–441.

9. Smith RA, Cokkinides V, Eyre HJ: American Cancer Society guidelines for the early detection of cancer, 2006. Cancer J Clin 2006; 56(1): 11–25.

10. US Preventive Services Task Force: Screening for colorectal cancer: recommendation and rationale. Ann Intern Med 2002; 137(2): 129–131.

11. Jeter JM, Kohlmann W, Gruber SB: Genetics of colorectal cancer. Oncology 2006; 20: 269–289.

12. Jimbo M, Nease DE, Ruffin MT, et al: Information technology and cancer prevention. CA Cancer J Clin 2006; 56: 26–36.

13. Tsao AS, Kim ES, Hong WK: Chemoprevention of cancer. Cancer J Clin 2004; 54: 150–180.

14. Janne PA, Mayer RJ: Chemoprevention of colorectal cancer. N Engl J Med 2000; 342(26): 1960–1968.

15. Kelloff GJ, Lippman SM, Dannenberg AJ, et al: Progress in chemoprevention drug development: the promise of molecular biomarkers for prevention of intraepithelial neoplasia and cancer – a plan to move forward. Clin Cancer Res 2006; 12(12): 3661–3697.

16. Hanahan D, Weinberg RA: The hallmarks of cancer. Cell 2000; 100: 57–70.

17. Chen Y, Hunter DJ: Molecular epidemiology of cancer. Cancer J Clin 2005; 55(1): 45–54.

18. Ramaswamy S, Golub TR: DNA microarrays in clinical oncology. J Clin Oncol 2002; 20(7): 1932–1941.

19. Quackenbush J: Microarray analysis and tumor classification. N Engl J Med 2006; 354: 2463–2472.

20. Geho DH, Petricoin EF, Liotta LA: Blasting into the microworld of tissue proteomics: a new window on cancer. Clin Cancer Research 2004; 10: 825–827.

21. Smith L, Lind MJ, Welham KJ, et al: Cancer proteomics and its application to discovery of therapy response markers in human cancer. Cancer 2006; 107(2): 232–241.

22. Herbst RS, Bajorin DF, Bleiberg H, et al: Clinical cancer advances 2005: major research advances in cancer treatment, prevention, and screening – a report from the American Society of Clinical Oncology. J Clin Oncol 2006; 24(1): 190–205.

23. Giantonio BJ, Catalano PJ, et al: High-dose bevacizumab improves survival when combined with FOLFOX4 in previously treated advanced colorectal cancer: results from the Eastern Cooperative Oncology Group (ECOG) study E3200. Proc Am Soc Clin Oncol 2005; 24: 2a.

24. Wilson RH: Novel therapeutic developments other than EGFR and VEGF inhibition in colorectal cancer. Oncologist 2006; 11(9): 1018–1024.

25. Engstrom PF, Benson AB 3rd, Chen YJ, et al: The NCCN colon cancer clinical practice guidelines. J Natl Compr Canc Netw 2005; 3: 468–491.

2

The role of molecular probes and other markers in the diagnosis and characterization of malignancy

Tad Wieczorek and Janina A. Longtine

Histopathological assessment is still the cornerstone in the diagnosis, classification and grading of malignancies. Light microscopic evaluation augmented by histochemical stains is sufficient in the majority of cases to provide adequate information for diagnosis and prognostication. However, it is limited by subjectivity and imprecision in the evaluation of poorly differentiated malignancies, tumours of unknown primary origin and unusual neoplasms. In an era of increasingly sophisticated therapeutic protocols (which sometimes target the molecular events leading to cancer) and the need to maximize information gained from minimally invasive samples (such as core biopsy or fine-needle aspiration), ancillary techniques have been developed to increase the specificity and reproducibility of diagnosis. These rely on cell-specific antigen expression and, more importantly, tumour-specific genetic changes that provide diagnostic, prognostic and/or therapeutic information.

In most instances, the advent of monoclonal antibodies directed against cellular proteins, coupled with the immunoperoxidase technique, has superseded direct ultrastructural evaluation in allowing more accurate designation of the epithelial, mesenchymal, haematolymphoid, neuroendocrine or glial origin of neoplasms. A cardinal example is immunolocalization of cytoskeletal intermediate filaments, which are differentially expressed in different cell types. Table 2.1 lists the intermediate filaments most useful in determining the cell lineage of tumours. The cytokeratins are a complex family of polypeptides that are expressed in various combinations in different epithelial cell types. Antibodies to cytokeratin subtypes can sometimes be utilized to identify the epithelial origin of a metastatic carcinoma of unknown primary site. For example, the pattern of reactivity for cytokeratin 7 (54 kD), which is expressed in most glandular and ductal epithelium and transitional epithelium of the urinary tract, and for cytokeratin 20 (46 kD), which is more restricted in its expression, has been helpful in this regard.[1]

In addition to the intermediate filaments, other monoclonal antibodies to cellular or tumour antigens are available. In the past decade, advances in the technique of immunohistochemistry have allowed

Table 2.1 Cytoskeletal intermediate filaments

Cell type	Intermediate filaments	Molecular weight or subtype	Presence in tumour
Epithelial	Cytokeratins	40–67	Keratinizing and non-keratinizing carcinomas
Mesenchymal	Vimentin	58	Wide distribution: sarcomas, melanomas, many lymphomas, some carcinomas
Muscle	Desmin	53	Leiomyosarcomas, rhabdomyosarcomas
Glial astrocytes	Glial fibrillary acidic protein	51	Gliomas (including astrocytomas), ependymomas
Neurons	Neurofilament proteins	68, 160, 200	Neural tumours, neuroblastomas

consistent, reliable application in routinely processed surgical pathology specimens.[2] Antigen retrieval techniques (including proteolytic digestion and heat-induced antigen retrieval), sensitive detection systems, automation and a broad range of antibodies have all contributed to this advance. Table 2.2 lists a panel of antibodies that can be utilized in routine formalin-fixed paraffin-embedded tissue to diagnose poorly differentiated neoplasms. A differential diagnosis is generated by clinical and morphological features, which can then be further refined by the use of immunohistochemistry. It is important to realize that the majority of antibodies are not entirely specific in lineage determination, and "aberrant" staining patterns are observed. In addition, there is biological variation in poorly differentiated neoplasms resulting in variation in protein expression. Therefore, accuracy is enhanced by using a panel of antisera to determine lineage or primary site. One application of this principle is distinguishing between poorly differentiated adenocarcinoma and mesothelioma in pleural tumours. Table 2.3 demonstrates the differential immunoprofile.

While a panel of monoclonal markers greatly aids in the diagnosis of a particular cancer, three malignancies can be confirmed solely by demonstrating the presence of a highly specific protein. Papillary and

Table 2.2 Immunocytochemistry in the differential diagnosis of malignancies

Malignancy	Keratin	Chromo-granin/synaptophysin	S100	MART-1	LCA	OCT 3/4	SMA/desmin
Carcinoma	+	–	–/+	–	–	–	–
Germ cell	+/–*	–	–	–	–	+/–	–
Lymphoma	–	–	–	–	+	–	–
Melanoma	–	–	+	+/–	–	–	–
Neuroendocrine	+/–	+	–	–	–	–	–
Sarcoma**	–/+	–	–/+	–/+	–	–	+/–

+ positive   +/– mainly positive, occasionally negative
– negative   –/+ mainly negative, occasionally positive

* Keratin is usually negative in seminomas, but positive in non-seminomatous germ cell tumours

**Sarcomas are a heterogeneous family of neoplasms and immunohistochemical staining patterns depend on the specific histological subtype

MART-1, Melanoma antigen recognized by T cells 1
LCA, Leukocyte common antigen
OCT3/4, Organic cation transporter 3/4
SMA, Smooth muscle actin

Table 2.3 Antibody panel in the differential diagnosis of adenocarcinoma and mesothelioma

Malignancy	Keratin*	WT-1	CD15 (Leu-M1)	CEA
Adenocarcinoma	+	–	+	+
Mesothelioma	+	+	–	–

*Keratin positivity in the appropriate clinicopathological setting limits the differential diagnosis to adenocarcinoma and mesothelioma

+ positive   – negative
CEA, carcinoembryonic antigen

follicular thyroid carcinomas are characterized by immunoreactivity to thyroglobulin, prostate carcinoma by detection of prostate-specific antigen, and breast carcinoma by a positive reaction for gross cystic disease fluid protein, which is present in approximately 50–70% of cases. It is noteworthy that the latter protein is also present in the rare apocrine gland carcinoma. Other antibodies which are not tissue-specific markers but useful in antibody panels include TTF-1 for pulmonary adenocarcinoma, RCC antigen for renal cell carcinoma, CD117 (c-kit) for gastrointestinal stromal tumours and CD31 (platelet endothelial cell adhesion molecule) for vascular endothelial neoplasms. Immunostains are also helpful in the delineation of normal tissue architecture and its abrogation in neoplasia. For example, immunostaining for p63 (a nuclear antigen expressed in myoepithelial cells of the breast and basal cells of the prostate) aids in the detection of ductal/glandular structures without the normal myoepithelial framework, the hallmark of invasive neoplasia.

While the cellular proteins expressed in particular types of neoplasia are fundamental to their diagnostic characterization, somatic mutations (i.e. mutations that occur in the genes of non-germline tissues) are central to the development of cancer. A series of different mutations in critical genes is probably necessary for malignant transformation to occur. The mutations may be deletions, duplications, point mutations and/or chromosomal translocations in the DNA of the tumour precursor cell. The mutations affect regulation of the cell cycle, differentiation, apoptosis, or cell–cell and cell–matrix interactions. Different neoplasms have different combinations of genetic alterations, which lead to clonal proliferations of cells. These genetic alterations, although fundamental in tumour biology, can also be used as diagnostic or prognostic markers for malignancies. This is best characterized in lymphomas and leukaemias where specific genetic translocations result in the production of chimeric mRNA and novel proteins. These translocations are the *sine qua non* for the classification of some leukaemias, such as the Philadelphia chromosome t(9;22)(q34;q11) for chronic myelogenous leukaemia and t(15;17)(q22;q11-21) for acute promyelocytic leukaemia.[3] Single nucleotide mutations may also be important in haematopoietic neoplasia; for example the *JAK2* V617F mutation is frequently present in chronic myeloproliferative disorders.[4] While genetic alterations in carcinomas are more complex than single point mutations or chromosome translocations, simple chromosomal translocations also commonly occur in (and characterize) soft tissue tumours.[5,6]

A global assessment of structural cytogenetic changes in a neoplasm is provided by full karyotypic analysis, which requires fresh, viable tumour. By contrast, fluorescence *in situ* hybridization (FISH) is a more targeted approach that can be performed on interphase nuclei obtained from frozen or fixed paraffin-embedded tissue and can identify specific characteristic cytogenetic abnormalities as an adjunct to tumour diagnosis. For example, FISH probes that flank the *EWS* gene region show a "split apart" signal when an *EWS* rearrangement is present, as in Ewing's sarcoma (see Figure 2.1). In addition, many of the characteristic cytogenetic abnormalities of neoplasms have been cloned and sequenced allowing for the utilization of molecular biology techniques such as Southern blot hybridization or, more commonly, the polymerase chain reaction (PCR). These techniques utilize fresh or frozen tumour, or even fixed, embedded tissue (with PCR), and improve diagnoses by identifying the characteristic chromosomal translocations of malignancies at the molecular level. With PCR, a specific translocation can be detected in as little as 1 in 100,000 or 1 in 1,000,000 cells as compared with 1 in 100 for FISH analysis. Thus, PCR provides a sensitive method for diagnosis and for monitoring response to therapy. For example, the t(9;22)(q34:q11) of chronic myelogenous leukaemia juxtaposes the *BCR* and *ABL1* genes resulting in a unique chimeric mRNA that can be detected by a quantitative real-time RT-PCR technique. Peripheral blood cell RNA is converted to cDNA by reverse transcription (RT). The resultant *BCR-ABL1* cDNA is quantified by monitoring fluorescently labelled oligonucleotide probes that specifically hybridize with the target during each cycle of PCR amplification (see Figure 2.2). Clinical trials with the tyrosine kinase inhibitor imatinib

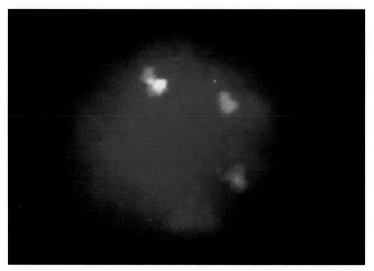

Fig. 2.1 Fluorescence *in situ* hybridization (FISH) on a sample obtained by fine-needle aspiration shows an interphase nucleus with red and green probes flanking each of two copies of the *EWS* gene, demonstrating one fused and one split signal. The split signal indicates rearrangement of the *EWS* gene region. (Courtesy of Dr. Paola Dal Cin, Cytogenetics Laboratory, Brigham and Women's Hospital.)

Colorectal Cancer

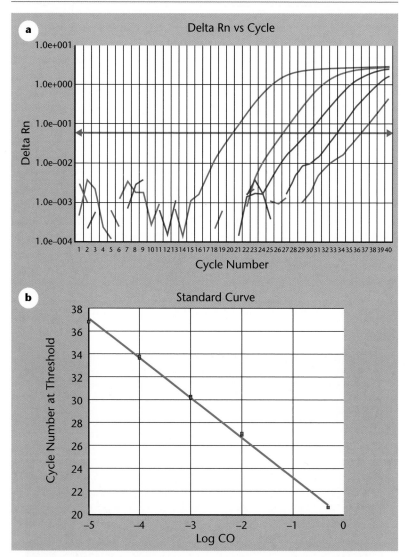

Fig. 2.2 (a) "Taq-Man™" (Applied Biosystems) quantitative RT-PCR results for dilutions (1:1,10^{-2}, 10^{-3}, 10^{-4}, 10^{-5}) of K562 cell line RNA which express chimeric *BCR-ABL1* mRNA. After approximately 15 cycles of PCR, the sample with the most *BCR-ABL1* mRNA (1:1) enters the linear phase of exponential amplification as measured by fluorescence accumulation monitored in real time. Samples with less target require more PCR cycles to reach the exponential phase. (b) For quantitation, a standard curve is generated plotting the PCR cycle number at threshold (red line in middle of exponential phase) against log concentration of target. Unknown samples can be quantified by plotting against the standard curve.

defined a target of a minimal residual level of *BCR-ABL1* RNA transcripts that is associated with progression-free survival (see Figure 2.3).[7,8] Rising levels of *BCR-ABL1* mRNA in patients on tyrosine kinase inhibitors or status post transplantation are indicative of a molecular relapse and the need for alternate or additional therapy. Southern blot hybridization or PCR can also identify clonal rearrangements of the immunoglobulin or T-cell receptor genes as an adjunct to the diagnosis of lymphoma or lymphoid leukaemias (see Figure 2.4).

Genetic analysis of neoplasms may also provide prognostic information, such as identifying the *BCR-ABL1* rearrangement in Philadelphia chromosome-positive acute lymphoblastic leukaemia (ALL) or *N-MYC* amplification in neuroblastoma. In addition, genetic analysis is playing an increasing role in therapeutic planning, as therapies tailored to specific genetic "lesions" are developed. Examples of such lesions include *HER2* amplification in breast cancer[9] and the epidermal growth factor receptor gene (*EGFR*) mutation in lung cancer.[10,11] These genetic lesions

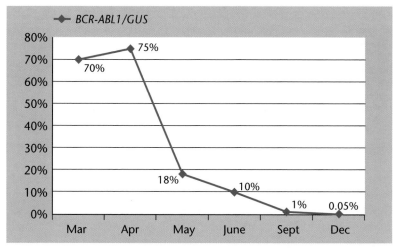

Fig. 2.3 Timeline of response to the tyrosine kinase inhibitor imatinib as monitored by real-time RT-PCR analysis of *BCR-ABL1* mRNA expressed as a ratio to the normalizing gene, *GUS*. Patients who achieve a 3-log reduction of transcript level by 12 months of therapy have a negligible risk of disease progression in the following 12 months.[8]

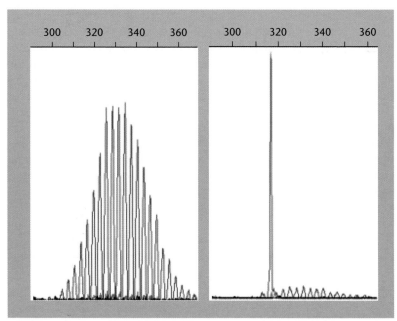

Fig. 2.4 Polymerase chain reaction (PCR) amplification of the immunoglobulin heavy chain (IgH) gene with primers to the variable and joining regions that flank the unique IgH gene rearrangement of B-cells. B-cell IgH rearrangements differ by size and sequence. Fluorescent primers are incorporated into the PCR product, which are then analyzed by capillary gel electrophoresis. (**a**) The Gaussian distribution of a polyclonal population of B cells. (**b**) A dominant peak of 318 bp representing a monoclonal population in a B-cell lymphoma.

may be detected either by evaluation of aberrant protein expression (as in immunohistochemical detection of membranous overexpression of HER2 oncoprotein in breast cancer), by gene amplification (as in FISH analysis of *HER2*), or by molecular testing (as in *EGFR* point or small deletion mutation analysis in lung cancer, see Figure 2.5). Quantification of the expression levels of large numbers of genes in specific types of neoplasia by oligonucleotide chips or cDNA microarrays, "expression profiling", has led to the identification of subsets of genes that provide prognostic information, such as in diffuse large B-cell lymphoma (see Figure 2.6).[12] It has even become feasible to measure the expression level of multiple genes (by RT-PCR) in routinely prepared, paraffin-embedded tumour samples, as in the multigene assay to

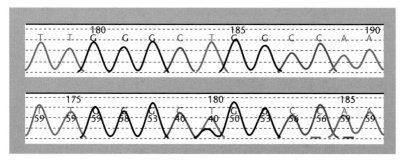

Fig. 2.5 Lung adenocarcinoma DNA sequence analysis of exon 21 of the *EGFR* receptor gene. The top row shows normal or wildtype exon sequence. The bottom row shows the heterozygous T to C point mutation, which characterizes the L858R mutation, a common mutation in carcinomas responsive to tyrosine kinase inhibitors.

predict recurrence of tamoxifen-treated, node-negative breast cancer.[13] This assay measures the expression level of genes involved in key aspects of tumour biology such as proliferation, invasion and oestrogen response and its quantitative result has potential application in therapeutic planning. As key genes (and hence proteins) are identified by expression profiling, expression can be assayed by routine immunohistochemistry. An important and practical example of this strategy was the development of a specific antibody to P504S (AMACR/racemase), a protein product strongly expressed in prostatic adenocarcinoma and prostatic intraepithelial neoplasia, but typically not in benign prostatic epithelium.[14] This immunostain is therefore useful in supporting a diagnosis of prostatic adenocarcinoma in cases where the morphological findings are subtle – as in the diagnosis of minimal adenocarcinoma on needle biopsy.

The genetics of cancer also extends to inherited predisposition to neoplasms described in a number of families.[15] These syndromes include germline mutations of tumour suppressor genes, such as familial retinoblastoma, and mutations of DNA repair genes as in ataxia-telangectasia or hereditary non-polyposis colon cancer. Some of these are listed in Table 2.4.

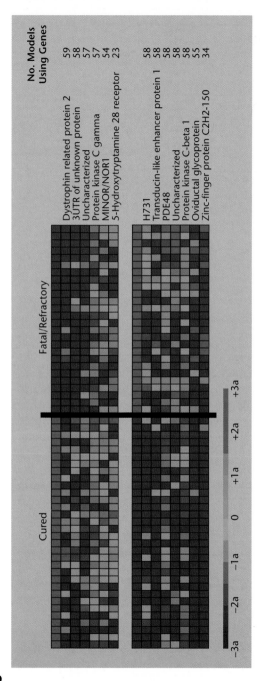

Fig. 2.6 Genes included in the DLBCL outcome model. Genes expressed at higher levels in cured disease are listed on top and those that were more abundant in fatal disease are shown on the bottom. Red indicates high expression; blue, low expression. Colour scale at bottom indicates relative expression in standard deviations from the mean. Each column is a sample, each row is a gene. Expression profiles of the 32 cured DLBCLs are on the left; profiles of the fatal/refractory tumours are on the right. Models with the highest accuracy were obtained using 13 genes. Reproduced by permission from Macmillan Publishers Ltd: Nature Medicine. Shipp M, Ross K, Tamayo P, et al: Diffuse large B-cell lymphoma outcome prediction by gene expression profiling and supervised machine learning. Nature Med 2002; 8: 68–74. © 2002.

Table 2.4 Examples of inherited syndromes predisposing to cancer

Syndrome	Chromosome locus	Gene
Ataxia-telangiactasia	11q22	*ATM*
Hereditary breast/ovarian cancer	17q21	*BRCA1*
	13q12	*BRCA2*
Familial adenomatous polyposis	5q21-q22	*APC*
Familial retinoblastoma	13q14	*RB1*
Hereditary non-polyposis colorectal cancer (Lynch syndrome)	2p22-p21	*MSH2*
	3p21	*MLH1*
	2q31-q33	*PMS1*
	7p22	*PMS2*
Li-Fraumeni	17p13	*TP53*
Multiple endocrine neoplasia, Type 1	11q13	*MEN1*
Multiple endocrine neoplasia, Type 2	10q11.2	*RET*
Neurofibromatosis, Type 1	17q11	*NF1*
Neurofibromatosis, Type 2	22q12	*NF2*
von Hippel-Lindau disease	3p26-p25	*VHL*

REFERENCES

1. Chu P, Wu E, Weiss LM: Cytokeratin 7 and cytokeratin 20 expression in epithelial neoplasms: a survey of 435 cases. Mod Pathol 2000; 13(9): 962–971.
2. Chan JKC: Advances in immunohistochemistry: Impact on surgical pathology practice. Seminars Diagn Pathol 2000; 17: 170–177.
3. Jaffe ES, Stein HN, Vardiman JW, eds: World Health Organization Classification of Tumours, Pathology and Genetics of Tumours of Haematopoietic and Lymphoid Tissues. IARC Press, Lyon, 2001.
4. Percy MJ, McMullin MF: The V617F JAK2 mutation and the myeloproliferative disorders. Hematol Oncol 2005; 23(3-4): 91–93.
5. Sandberg AA: Cytogenetics and molecular genetics of bone and soft-tissue tumors. Am J Med Genet 2002; 115(3): 189–193.
6. Antonescu CR: The role of genetic testing in soft tissue sarcoma. Histopathology 2006; 48(1): 13–21.
7. O'Brien SG, Guilhot F, Larson RA, et al: Imatinib compared with interferon and low-dose cytarabine for newly diagnosed chronic-phase chronic myeloid leukemia. N Engl J Med 2003; 348: 994–1004.
8. Hughes TP, Kaeda J, Branford S, et al: Frequency of major molecular responses to imatinib or interferon alfa plus cytarabine in newly diagnosed chronic myeloid leukemia. N Engl J Med 2003; 349: 1423–1432.

9. Slamon DJ, Leyland-Jones B, Shak S, et al: Use of chemotherapy plus a monoclonal antibody against HER2 for metastatic breast cancer that overexpresses HER2. N Engl J Med 2001; 344: 783–792.

10. Lynch TJ, Bell DW, Sordella R, et al: Activating mutations in the epidermal growth factor receptor underlying responsiveness of non-small-cell lung cancer to gefitinib. N Engl J Med 2004; 350: 2129–2139.

11. Paez JG, Janne PA, Lee JC, et al: EGFR mutations in lung cancer: correlation with clinical response to gefitinib therapy. Science 2004; 304: 1497–1500.

12. Shipp M, Ross K, Tamayo P, et al: Diffuse large B-cell lymphoma outcome prediction by gene expression profiling and supervised machine learning. Nature Med 2002; 8: 68–74.

13. Paik S, Shak S, Tang G, et al: A multigene assay to predict recurrence of tamoxifen-treated, node-negative breast cancer. N Engl J Med 2004; 351: 2817–2826.

14. Beach R, Gown AM, De Peralta-Venturina MN, et al: P504S immunohistochemical detection in 405 prostatic specimens including 376 18-gauge needle biopsies. Am J Surg Pathol 2002; 26(12): 1588–1596.

15. Scriver CR, Beaudet AL, Sly WS, Valle D, eds: Metabolic and Molecular Bases of Inherited Disease, 8th edn. McGraw-Hill, New York, 2001.

Colorectal cancer: epidemiology, histology, diagnosis and staging

3

Matthew H. Kulke, Jerrold R. Turner, Jeffrey Meyerhardt

Colorectal cancer (CRC) is the fourth most common malignancy and the second most frequent cause of cancer-related death in the US. In 2007, an estimated 153,760 cases of CRC will be diagnosed and 52,180 people will die from this disease.[1] Worldwide, CRC is the fourth most commonly diagnosed malignancy, with an estimated 1,023,152 new cases and 528,978 deaths each year.[2] Approximately 70% of these cancers will arise in the colon, while 30% will occur in the rectum. Overall mortality from CRC has declined progressively in the past two decades, partially as a result of detection of disease at an earlier stage, and more effective treatments, particularly adjuvant therapy.

RISK FACTORS

The incidence of colon cancer is highest in industrialized areas such as the US and Europe (see Figure 3.2). As a result, epidemiological studies have focused on identifying factors prevalent in these populations that relatively increase and decrease one's risk of developing CRC. In addition to family history and certain medical conditions, a host of dietary and lifestyle factors have been consistently shown to modify this risk (see Table 3.1).

Table 3.1 Risk factors for developing colorectal cancer

Increase risk	Decrease risk	Risk relationship uncertain
Family history	Screening	Cholesterol-lowering agents (statins)
Obesity	Physical activity	Fibre
Inflammatory bowel disease	Aspirin	Fruits and vegetables
Diabetes	Calcium / vitamin D	
High intake of red meat	Postmenopausal hormones	
Alcohol	Folate intake	
Tobacco smoking		

FAMILY HISTORY

Up to 25% of all patients with CRC have a family history of the disease.[3] Several hereditary syndromes are associated with an increased risk for colon cancer. Familial adenomatous polyposis (FAP) is a rare autosomal dominant condition that is characterized by the development of numerous polyps throughout the colon (see Figures 3.15–3.18).[4] Virtually all patients with FAP will develop colon cancer by age 40 unless prophylactic colectomy is performed. FAP is caused by germline mutations in the tumour suppressor gene *APC*. Variants of FAP include Gardner's syn-

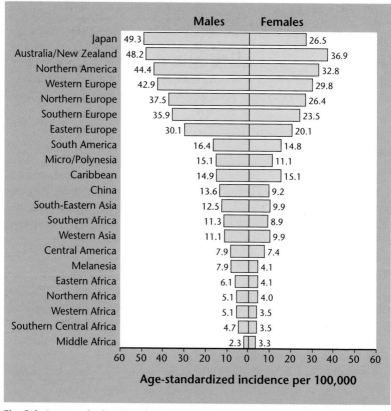

Fig. 3.1 Age-standardized incidence rates for colorectal cancer. Data shown per 100,000 by sex. Reproduced with permission from Parkin DM, Bray F, Ferlay J, Pisani P: Global Cancer Statistics, 2002. CA Cancer J Clin 2005; 55: 74–108.

drome (in which prominent extraintestinal lesions like desmoid tumours and sebaceous or epidermoid cysts are seen in addition to extensive polyposis) and Turcot's syndrome (brain tumours, particularly medulloblastomas, in addition to colonic tumours). The importance of *APC* is emphasized by the observation that it is mutated in colon tumours (but not the germ line) of some patients with sporadic (i.e. non-hereditary) colon cancer.

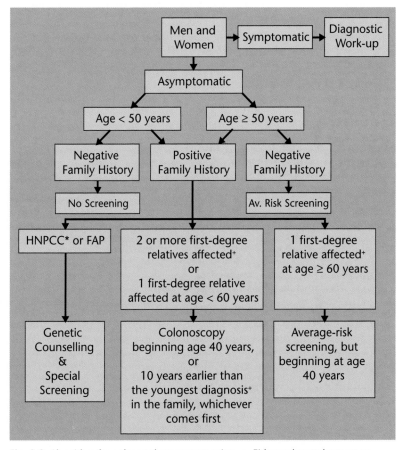

Fig. 3.2 Algorithm for colorectal cancer screening. +, Either colorectal cancer or adenomatous polyp; *, HNPCC, hereditary non-polyposis colorectal cancer; FAP, familial adenomatous polyposis. Reproduced with permission from Winawer S, Fletcher R, Rex D, et al: Colorectal cancer screening and surveillance: Clinical guidelines and rationale—Update based on new evidence. Gastroenterology 2003; 124(2): 544–560.

Hereditary non-polyposis colon cancer (HNPCC), another inherited syndrome, is characterized by the early onset of colon cancer, often involving the right side of the colon, and typically occurring in the absence of numerous colonic polyps.[5] Several germline defects responsible for HNPCC have been identified; the most common of these are mutations in *hMLH1* and *hMSH2*. These genes are essential components of a nucleotide mismatch repair system. HNPCC is also associated with the development of extracolonic tumours, including malignancies of the endometrium, ovary, stomach and small bowel. Genetic screening for individuals at risk for HNPCC is available.

In addition to familial syndromes, a family or personal history of CRC or adenomatous polyps increases one's risk of developing CRC.[3] This risk is modified by number of family members affected and age of diagnosis of family members, particularly first-degree relatives.

ASSOCIATED DISEASES

Patients with inflammatory bowel disease (IBD) have an increased risk of CRC that can be up to 10 fold higher than the general population (see Figures 3.19–3.21).[6,7] While initial observations suggested such a risk was limited to patients with ulcerative colitis, recent evidence also implicates Crohn's disease as a risk factor.[8] Extent of disease involvement of the colon and rectum and duration of disease are the main determinants of the increased risk. In general, patients with ulcerative colitis do not have an appreciable increase in risk until about 8–10 years from time of diagnosis of IBD.

Diabetes mellitus has also been associated with a risk of CRC.[9] The potential mechanism is related to insulin and insulin-like growth factor (IGF), stimulants of colonic cell growth. Case-control and cohort studies have suggested that diabetic patients have a 1.3–1.5 fold increased risk of CRC, compared with non-diabetics. However, given the prevalence of diabetes, such a relative risk is clinically significant.

Individuals with acromegaly have a 2.5 fold increased risk of CRC.[10,11] Though the mechanism of this increased risk is not entirely clear, the elevated levels of growth factor and IGF-1 characteristic of acromegaly probably stimulate colonic mucosa proliferation.

DIETARY AND LIFESTYLE FACTORS

Epidemiology studies have identified dietary factors that contribute to the risk of developing CRC.[12] Prospective cohort studies link high intake of red meat,[13-15] low intake of folic acid,[16] and decreased calcium and vitamin D[17-19] to increased risk of developing CRC. Fibre intake and fruit and vegetables have been studied extensively as risk factors, though the majority of studies show little or no association except in the case of very low intake of these dietary factors.[20-25]

Obesity and physical activity have consistently been shown to influence the risk of CRC. Increasing body mass index and lower levels of physical activity increase the risk of developing CRC up to 2 fold.[26-30] Recent hypotheses have linked physical activity, obesity and adipose distribution to circulating insulin and free IGF-1.[31-33]

An association between alcohol consumption and an increased risk of CRC has been observed in several studies. A pooled analysis of eight cohort studies estimated a 40% increased risk of CRC in those whose alcohol consumption exceeded 45 g per day. The amount of alcohol in a 12 ounce (0.75 pints, 355 ml) beer, 4 ounce (0.25 pint, 118 ml) glass of wine, and 1.5 ounce (44 ml) shot of 80-proof liquor was estimated to be 13, 11 and 14 g, respectively. Cigarette smoking has been associated both with increased incidence of and mortality from CRC.[34,35]

MEDICATIONS AND CRC

Preclinical,[36-38] epidemiological,[39-41] and intervention studies[42-46] support a protective effect of aspirin, NSAIDs and selective cyclo-oxygenase-2 (COX-2) inhibitors on the risk of CRC and adenomas. Recently, the use of 3-hydroxy-3-methylglutaryl coenzyme A reductase inhibitors, commonly known as statins, have been tested as to whether they provide a protective effect against CRC development.[47,48] To date, studies have been mixed and the potential benefit remains unclear.

HISTOLOGY AND STAGING

HISTOLOGY

Over 98% of cancers of the large bowel are adenocarcinomas. Characteristic subgroups include mucinous or colloid tumours and signet ring cell tumours. Adenocarcinomas are classified as well, moderately or poorly differentiated, each category having a distinct prognostic implication. Most colorectal carcinomas originate from adenomatous polyps (see Table 3.2). Pathologically, progression from early adenomatous proliferations through adenomatous polyp, high-grade dysplasia and, ultimately, invasive carcinoma occurs as a continuum. This progression coincides with the accumulation of genetic alterations within the neoplasm as originally described by Drs Eric Fearon and Bert Vogelstein.[49] These alterations include mutations of tumour suppressor genes, e.g. *p53*, *DCC* and *APC*, as well as activation and/or overexpression of oncogenes, e.g. c-*myc* and k-*ras*. While the order of occurrence of these genetic changes may vary, the quantitative accumulation of defects correlates with biological and histological parameters of neoplastic progression, suggesting a multistep model of tumorigenesis. The majority of bowel cancers arise in the rectum and sigmoid colon; however, recent studies show that, for unknown reasons, the proportion of cancers arising in the rectum is decreasing, whereas the percentage of those originating in the caecum and ascending colon is increasing (see Figure 3.3). The remaining 2% of CRCs consist of lymphomas, leiomyosarcomas and miscellaneous tumours.

Table 3.2 Classification of colonic polyps

Type	Histopathology	Associated diseases
Neoplastic	Adenoma	None (sporadic)
	tubular adenoma	Familial adenomatous polyposis
	tubulovillous adenoma	Gardner's syndrome
	villous adenoma	Turcot syndrome
Non-neoplastic	Hyperplastic polyp	None (sporadic)
		Hyperplastic polyposis
	Hamartomatous polyp	None (sporadic)
		Peutz–Jeghers syndrome
	Inflammatory fibroid polyp	None (sporadic)
	Inflammatory pseudopolyp	Ulcerative colitis, Crohn's disease
		Ischaemic colitis
		Infection (amoebiasis, schistosomiasis)
		Ulceration
	Juvenile polyp	None (sporadic)
		Juvenile polyposis syndrome
		Cronkhite-Canada syndrome
	Lymphoid polyp	None (incidental, reactive)
		Lymphoid polyposis

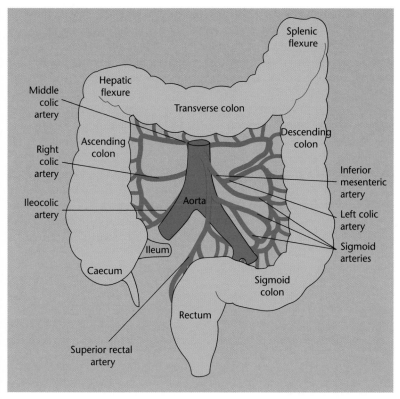

Fig. 3.3 Anatomical segments and vascular supply of the colon.

STAGING OF CRCs

CRCs are generally staged at the time of surgery (see Figures 3.22 and 3.23). Computed tomography (CT) scans of the abdomen and pelvis and chest radiographs are usually also performed to evaluate for metastatic disease. Bone scans are not routinely carried out in the absence of bone pain, due to a low incidence of bone metastases. Extension of primary rectal cancers into adjacent soft tissues can often be assessed by pelvic magnetic resonanse imaging (MRI) or endorectal ultrasound. Positron emission tomography (PET) scans are utilized to further evaluate abnormalities detected on CT scans but not routinely performed in the initial staging of CRCs. In addition, they are useful to evaluate patients that may have a metastectomy performed to rule out other distant metastases.

Several systems have been employed in staging CRC. The initial staging system was introduced by Dukes and subsequently modified by Kirklin and colleagues, Astler and Coller, and others. These classifications were based on three prognostic variables: depth of tumour invasion through the bowel wall, regional lymph node involvement and distant metastases. Unlike other cancers, the size of the primary colon carcinoma does not in itself affect prognosis. These systems have largely been replaced by the more universal cancer TNM (tumour, node, metastases) staging system. The 6th edition of the American Joint Commission on Cancer revised the TNM staging classification,[50] where new subcategories of stage II and III CRC are included to differentiate tumours based on the extent of invasion through the bowel wall and the number of involved lymph nodes (1–3 vs. 4 or more). As recent studies have shown, the 5-year survival rate for each stage of disease, except for stage IV, has improved. The reasons for this trend may not necessarily be related to improvements in early detection and in surgical technique but rather to more thorough and accurate staging.

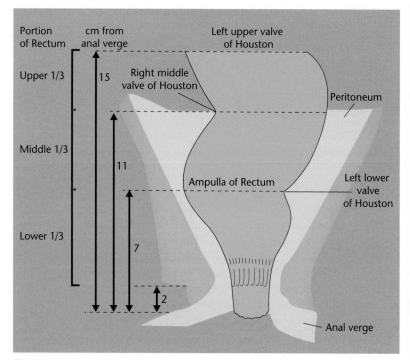

Fig. 3.4 Anatomy of the rectum.

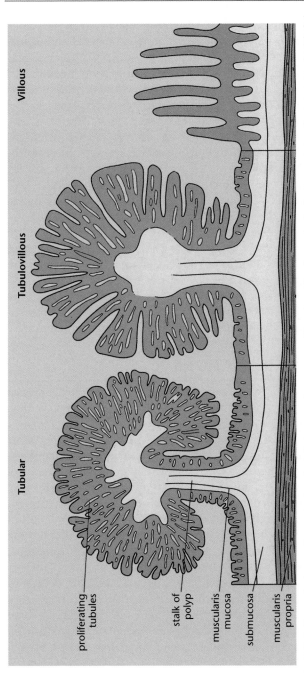

Fig. 3.5 Patterns of adenomatous colonic polyps. Polyps may be pedunculated (left, middle) or sessile (right). The surface epithelium of the stalk may be non-neoplastic (left) or adenomatous (middle). Polyps may be solitary or multiple; the presence of more than approximately 100 polyps suggests the diagnosis of familial adenomatous polyposis. Although they can arise at any site in the large bowel, the largest and more often symptomatic lesions tend to be situated in the left side of the colon. The diagnosis of adenoma requires the presence of epithelial dysplasia. These polyps are, therefore, premalignant neoplastic tissue. Factors believed to increase the risk of malignant change include large polyp size (particularly > 2 cm in diameter), severe epithelial dysplasia and villous architecture. Penetration of the muscularis mucosa by dysplastic epithelium, with invasion of the submucosa, is the distinguishing sign of invasive carcinoma.

Labels (left to right): Tubular, Tubulovillous, Villous

proliferating tubules

stalk of polyp

muscularis mucosa

submucosa

muscularis propria

CRCs spread by direct invasion, through lymphatic channels, along haematogenous routes and by implantation (see Table 3.3 and Figures 3.32 and 3.34). Spread of colon cancers through the portal venous circulation leads to liver metastases, which are present in about two-thirds of patients at autopsy. Cancers that originate below the peritoneal reflection (12–15 cm from the anal verge) are considered rectal cancers. The location of these lesions and the lymphatic drainage of this area necessitate special management decisions. Rectal cancers situated below the peritoneal reflection have a high rate of local recurrence. Cancers of the lower rectum may metastasize via the paravertebral plexus to supraclavicular nodes, lungs, bone and brain, without liver involvement.

Initial staging remains the most predictive prognostic factor for overall survival. Patients with stage I disease have >90% 5-year survival with surgery. Patients with stage II disease have 70–85% 5-year survival (dependent on extent of disease through bowel wall and existence of other prognostic features – clinical bowel obstruction, bowel perforation and poor differentiation give higher risk for recurrence). Patients with stage III disease have a variable 5-year survival of 35–70% (depending on the number of positive lymph nodes and presence of other high-risk features). Finally, patients with stage IV disease (metastastic) have less than 5% long-term survival.[1,51]

CLINICAL MANIFESTATIONS

Patients with cancer of the caecum and ascending colon usually present with anaemia caused by intermittent gastrointestinal bleeding. Obstruction is rare, because the bowel wall is more distensible and has a greater circumference than the descending colon. These cancers are often large and may be fungating or friable. Carcinomas of the transverse colon and either the hepatic or the splenic flexure, which account for about 10% of total cases, are somewhat less common than caecal neoplasms and much less common than rectosigmoid tumours. They frequently cause cramping pain, bleeding and sometimes obstruction or perforation. Large bowel obstruction is the most common complication of colon carcinoma and may lead to proximal ulceration or perforation. Obstruction is the principal reason why up to 30% of cases present as surgical emergencies. Other complications include iron deficiency anaemia, hypokalaemia (particularly associated with large villous rectal lesions) and intussusception in adults. Tumours of the sigmoid colon and rectum cancers usually cause changes in normal bowel habits, with tenesmus, decrease in stool calibre, secretion of mucus and haematochezia (see Figure 3.35).

CRC is usually initially diagnosed with colonoscopy. A full colonoscopy should be performed in all patients with CRC to rule out the possibility of second occult primary colon cancers, which occur in about 5% of patients. Surgical resection of the primary CRC is generally performed either with curative intent or, in patients with metastatic disease, as a palliative procedure to reduce the risk of obstruction and bleeding.

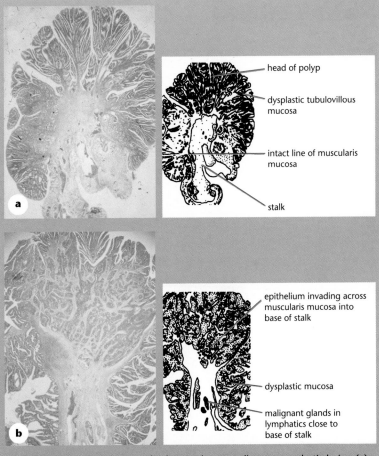

head of polyp

dysplastic tubulovillous mucosa

intact line of muscularis mucosa

stalk

epithelium invading across muscularis mucosa into base of stalk

dysplastic mucosa

malignant glands in lymphatics close to base of stalk

Fig. 3.6 Adenomatous lesions of colon. In the premalignant neoplastic lesion (**a**), the muscularis mucosa is intact, whereas in the malignant lesion (**b**) the muscularis is obviously invaded by malignant epithelium. Malignant glands in the lymphatics are seen close to the base of the stalk.

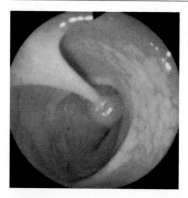

Fig. 3.7 Tubular adenoma. Endoscopy shows a pedunculated adenomatous polyp of the colon.

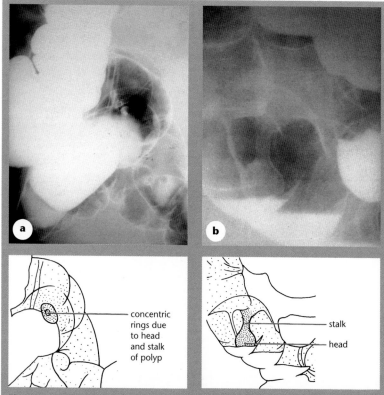

Fig. 3.8 Tubular adenoma. (**a**) Barium enema study shows a pedunculated polyp en face. The two rings formed by the polyp and the stalk are called the "target sign". (**b**) Lateral decubitus view confirms that the polyp is pedunculated.

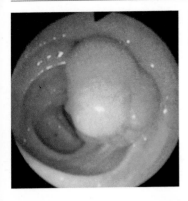

Fig. 3.9 Tubulovillous adenoma. Endoscopic view shows a moderate-sized sessile polyp. Several lobules are evident.

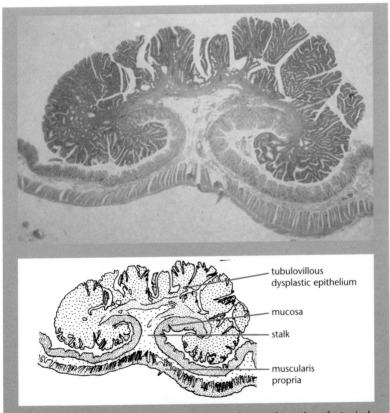

tubulovillous dysplastic epithelium

mucosa

stalk

muscularis propria

Fig. 3.10 Tubulovillous adenoma. Low-power microscopic section of a typical stalked lesion shows the closely packed dysplastic epithelial tubules, separated by lamina propria. The stalk is uninvolved and composed of submucosa and normal mucosa.

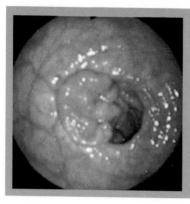

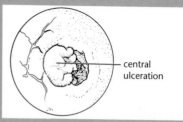

Fig. 3.11 Villous adenoma. Malignant rectal villous polyp. Endoscopy shows superficial central ulceration in this rectal polyp, suggestive of malignancy.

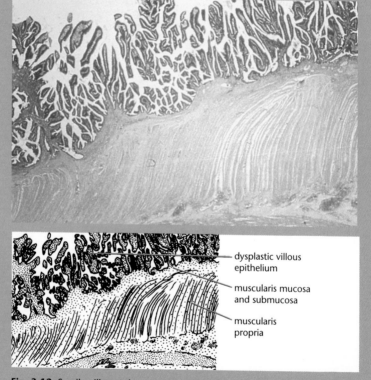

Fig. 3.12 Sessile villous adenoma. Histological section of a villous polyp demonstrates its sessile nature. Note the numerous finger-like villi, with dysplastic epithelium over a core of lamina propria, resting directly on the muscularis mucosa. No invasion is present.

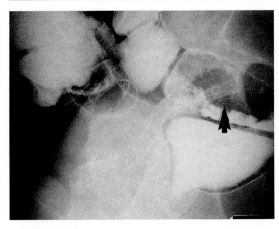

Fig. 3.13 Villous adenoma. A broad rectal lesion can be seen rising posteriorly (arrow). Histological examination revealed a villous adenoma. Tumours of this size have a high probability of malignancy and are too large and broad-based for endoscopic removal. Typical symptoms include copious, watery, mucus-containing diarrhoea, rectal bleeding and tenesmus.

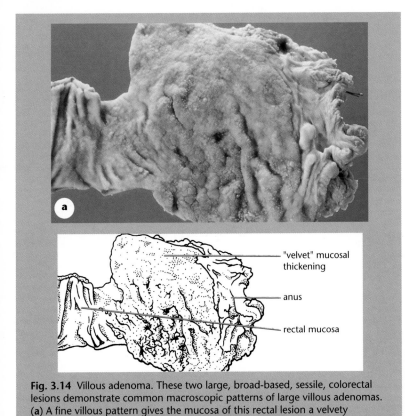

"velvet" mucosal thickening

anus

rectal mucosa

Fig. 3.14 Villous adenoma. These two large, broad-based, sessile, colorectal lesions demonstrate common macroscopic patterns of large villous adenomas. (a) A fine villous pattern gives the mucosa of this rectal lesion a velvety appearance. *continued*

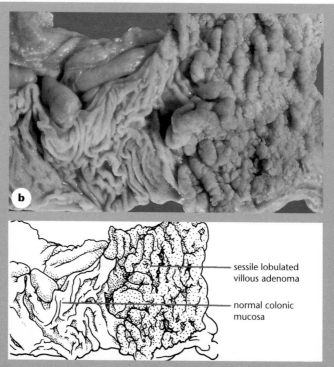

sessile lobulated
villous adenoma

normal colonic
mucosa

Fig. 3.14 *continued* This is in contrast to (**b**) the coarser, lobulated pattern seen in this colonic adenoma. The margins of both lesions are ill defined. Villous adenomas are most common in the rectum, where they tend to be larger and to show more severe dysplasia than tubular adenomas; they therefore more commonly progress to adenocarcinoma. Villous adenomas of the rectum sometimes secrete large amounts of potassium or albumin, giving rise to hypokalaemia or hypoalbuminaemia.

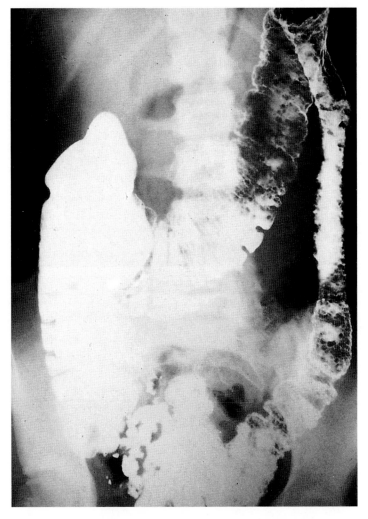

Fig. 3.15 Familial adenomatous polyposis. Barium enema study demonstrates multiple, small polyps throughout the colon.

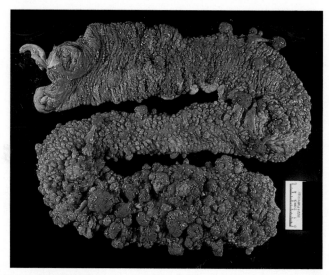

Fig. 3.16 Familial adenomatous polyposis, with innumerable adenomatous polyps, increasing in size and density from proximal (upper left) to distal (lower right). Microscopic section of one of the largest polyps (left) demonstrates a focal area of invasive adenocarcinoma (right) characterized by irregular, infiltrative gland architecture and an associated desmoplastic stroma.

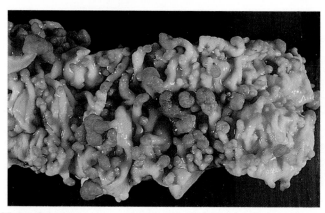

Fig. 3.17 Familial adenomatous polyposis. This disorder is marked by the development of hundreds of large bowel adenomas, as seen in this segment of large bowel, which is covered with adenomas of various sizes. It usually arises in the second and third decades.

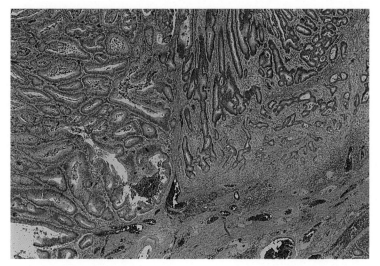

Fig. 3.18 Familial adenomatous polyposis (FAP). Section of colon shows innumerable polyps characteristic of FAP. If left untreated, the risk of colon cancer in such patients approaches 100% by the age of 40.

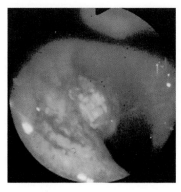

Fig. 3.19 Polypoid epithelial dysplasia in ulcerative colitis. Endoscopy reveals epithelial dysplasia with surrounding chronic active colitis in a patient who had ulcerative colitis for nearly 20 years. Histological examination showed high-grade mucosal dysplasia. The dysplasia is histologically identical to that seen in adenomatous polyps. However, in the setting of ulcerative colitis of >10 years duration, high-grade dysplasia is strongly associated with the development of invasive cancer and should prompt serious consideration of colectomy.

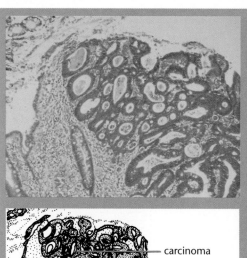

Fig. 3.20 Intramucosal carcinoma in ulcerative colitis. Frank intramucosal carcinoma is evident in this colon biopsy specimen from a patient with ulcerative colitis. The lesion infiltrates the lamina propria but does not extend beyond the muscularis mucosa. The tumour evolves through ascending grades of dysplasia in non-polypoid mucosa, as evidenced by the uninvolved mucosa at the left margin.

carcinoma

uninvolved mucosa

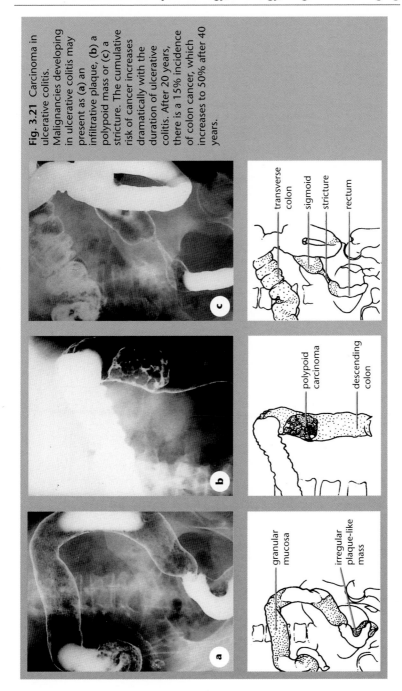

Fig. 3.21 Carcinoma in ulcerative colitis. Malignancies developing in ulcerative colitis may present as (a) an infiltrative plaque, (b) a polypoid mass or (c) a stricture. The cumulative risk of cancer increases dramatically with the duration of ulcerative colitis. After 20 years, there is a 15% incidence of colon cancer, which increases to 50% after 40 years.

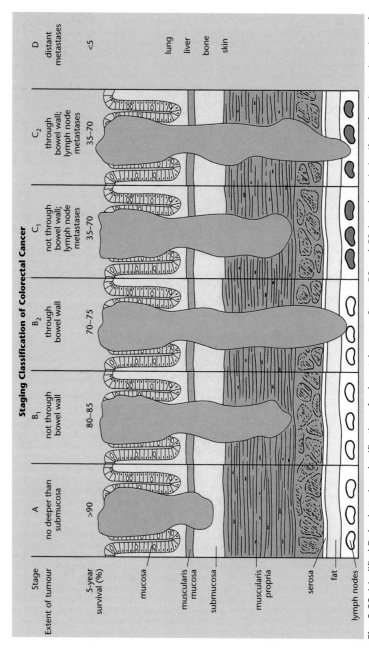

Staging Classification of Colorectal Cancer

Stage	A	B₁	B₂	C₁	C₂	D
Extent of tumour	no deeper than submucosa	not through bowel wall	through bowel wall	not through bowel wall; lymph node metastases	through bowel wall; lymph node metastases	distant metastases
5-year survival (%)	>90	80–85	70–75	35–70	35–70	<5

mucosa
muscularis mucosa
submucosa
muscularis propria
serosa
fat
lymph nodes

lung
liver
bone
skin

Fig. 3.22 Modified Dukes' staging classification of colorectal cancer. Stages B3 and C3 (not shown) signify perforation or invasion of contiguous organs or structures (T4). The TNM classification provides a more accurate staging system: Dukes B is a composite of better (T2N0) and worse (T3N0, T4N0) prognostic groups, as is Dukes C (TxN1 or TxN2).

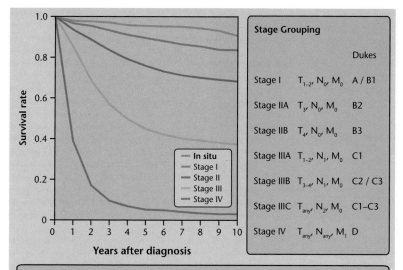

Stage Grouping		Dukes
Stage I	T_{1-2}, N_0, M_0	A / B1
Stage IIA	T_3, N_0, M_0	B2
Stage IIB	T_4, N_0, M_0	B3
Stage IIIA	T_{1-2}, N_1, M_0	C1
Stage IIIB	T_{3-4}, N_1, M_0	C2 / C3
Stage IIIC	T_{any}, N_2, M_0	C1–C3
Stage IV	T_{any}, N_{any}, M_1	D

Survival rate — Years after diagnosis

In situ
Stage I
Stage II
Stage III
Stage IV

Definition of TNM
The same classification is used for both clinical and pathological staging.

Primary Tumour (T)
TX Primary tumour cannot be assessed
T0 No evidence of primary tumour
Tis Carcinoma *in situ*: intraepithelial or invasion of lamina propria*
T1 Tumour invades submucosa
T2 Tumour invades muscularis propria
T3 Tumour invades through the muscularis propria into the subserosa, or into
    non-peritonealized pericolic or perirectal tissues
T4 Tumour directly invades other organs or structures, and/or perforates visceral peritoneum**

*Note: Tis includes cancer cells confined within the glandular basement membrane (intraepithelial) or lamina propria (intramucosal) with no extension through the muscularis mucosa into the submucosa.
**Note: Direct invasion in T4 includes invasion of other segments of the colorectum by way of the serosa, for example, invasion of the sigmoid colon by a carcinoma of the caecum.

Regional Lymph Nodes (N)
NX Regional lymph nodes cannot be assessed
N0 No regional lymph node metastasis
N1 Metastasis in 1 to 3 regional lymph nodes
N2 Metastasis in 4 or more regional lymph nodes

Distant Metastasis (M)
MX Distant metastasis cannot be assessed
M0 No distant metastasis
M1 Distant metastasis

Relative survival rates of patients with colon cancer according to the stage of disease. Rates based on 111,110 patients. Data taken from the Surveillance, Epidemiology and End Results Program of the National Cancer Institute for the years 1973–1987. Patients were staged according to the current TNM. Stage 0 (*in situ*) includes 4,841 patients; Stage II, 19,623; Stage II, 33,798; Stage III, 29,615; and Stage IV, 23,233.

Fig. 3.23 TNM staging of colorectal cancer.[50]

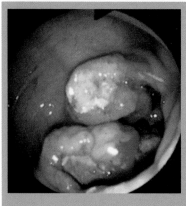

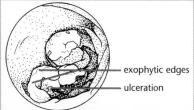

exophytic edges

ulceration

Fig. 3.24 Adenocarcinoma of caecum. Endoscopic view shows tumour presenting as a centrally excavated mass with exophytic overhanging edges. The ulceration is typically irregular, deep and grey or pink, with a necrotic appearance.

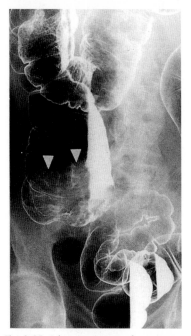

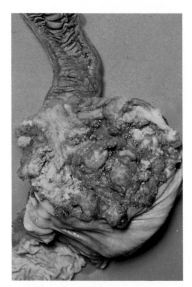

Fig. 3.25 Adenocarcinoma of caecum. Intestinal obstruction occurs late in the course of the disease. Although this lesion (arrows) is relatively large, there was no obstruction to retrograde filling of the ileum and no dilatation of the small intestine. Symptoms may include anaemia or dyspepsia and weight loss reminiscent of a benign or malignant gastric ulcer.

Fig. 3.26 Adenocarcinoma of caecum. Large, fungating tumours, as seen here, are a less common presentation of colorectal tumours; they predominate in the caecum.

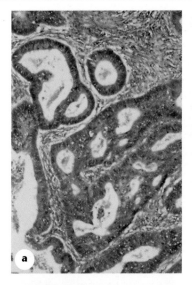

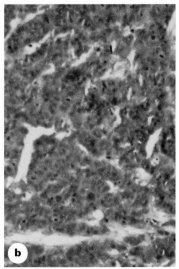

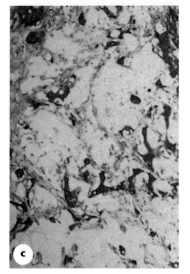

Fig. 3.27 Adenocarcinoma. (**a**) Moderately differentiated tumours are marked by gland (acinar) formation by malignant epithelium; there is considerable nuclear pleomorphism within individual cells. (**b**) In poorly differentiated lesions, sheets of malignant epithelial cells can be seen with little acinar formation. (**c**) The mucinous (colloid) variant exhibits nests of malignant epithelium in pools of mucin.

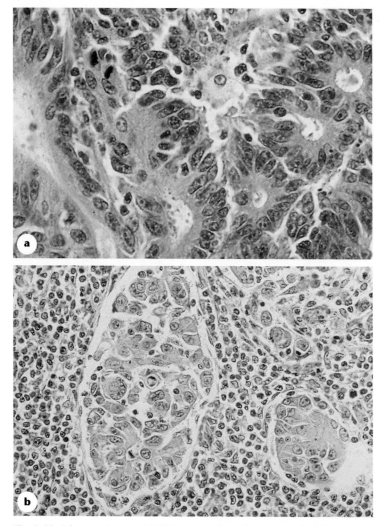

Fig. 3.28 Adenocarcinoma. (a) High-power view of a moderately differentiated tumour shows irregular and hyperchromatic nuclei, prominent nucleoli and several mitoses. (b) Metastases are evident in this lymph node biopsy.

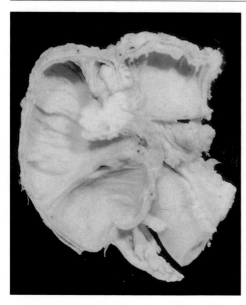

Fig. 3.29 Adenocarcinoma of ascending colon. This specimen is from a 57-year-old man who presented with a 1-year history of right upper quadrant abdominal pain. Examination revealed a tender mass beneath the right costal margin and barium enema film showed a tumour just proximal to the hepatic flexure. A right hemicolectomy was performed. The distal ileum, caecum and ascending colon have been opened to show an annular, stenosing neoplasm at the hepatic flexure; the bowel lumen has been reduced to a narrow cleft. Proximally, there is obvious dilatation of the intestine, with some associated muscle hypertrophy.

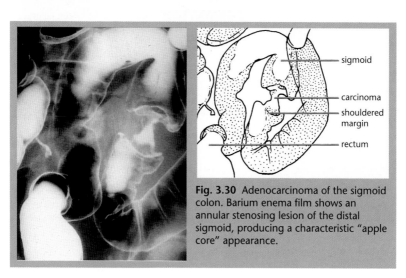

Fig. 3.30 Adenocarcinoma of the sigmoid colon. Barium enema film shows an annular stenosing lesion of the distal sigmoid, producing a characteristic "apple core" appearance.

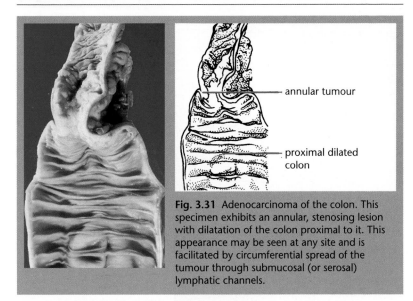

Fig. 3.31 Adenocarcinoma of the colon. This specimen exhibits an annular, stenosing lesion with dilatation of the colon proximal to it. This appearance may be seen at any site and is facilitated by circumferential spread of the tumour through submucosal (or serosal) lymphatic channels.

annular tumour

proximal dilated colon

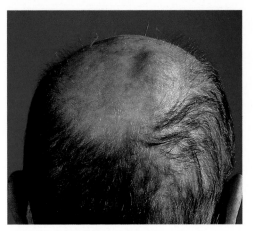

Fig. 3.32 Metastatic colon cancer. A 60-year-old man with previous colectomy for stage III colon cancer 4 years earlier developed a nodule on his posterior scalp. Biopsy was positive for poorly differentiated adenocarcinoma, similar to the original cancer. Carcinoembryonic antigen was elevated at 50 ng/ml. Subsequent studies showed multiple liver metastases. Skin metastases are not common, but have been reported in colon, pancreatic, breast and lung cancers as well as miscellaneous other malignancies.

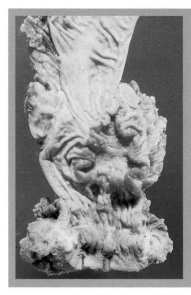

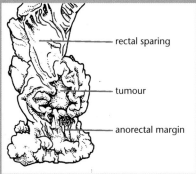

rectal sparing

tumour

anorectal margin

Fig. 3.33 Adenocarcinoma of the rectum. This lower rectal lesion demonstrates the most common macroscopic appearance of colorectal cancers as well-circumscribed lesions with raised edges and an ulcerated centre.

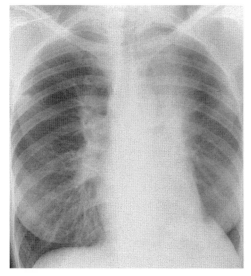

Fig. 3.34 Metastatic colorectal cancer. A 34-year-old woman with prior anterior-posterior resection for a stage II rectal cancer 3 years earlier presented with clinical features of superior vena cava (SVC) syndrome. Chest radiograph showed mediastinal adenopathy and atelectatic changes in the left upper lobe. Chest CT scan and nuclide flow studies (not shown) revealed tumour obstruction of the SVC. Mediastinoscopy was positive for adenocarcinoma with features similar to the original rectal carcinoma. Bronchoscopy showed no intrinsic lesions. Radiotherapy resulted in a partial remission. Liver metastases eventually occurred. Metastatic colorectal carcinoma may spread to the lungs and mediastinum and bypass the liver due to lymphatic spread via the paravertebral vascular channels of Batson as well as lower pelvic collaterals.

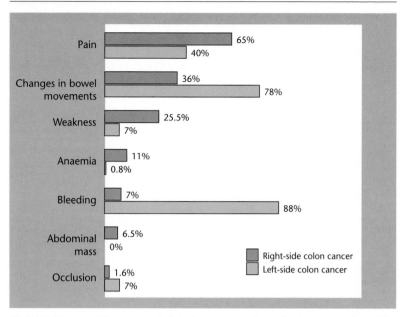

Fig 3.35 Compared frequency of clinical symptomatology of colon cancer (from 180 cancers). Adapted from Metman EH, Bertrand J, Bouleau PH: [Clinical and x-ray diagnosis of right colonic cancers]. Rev Prat 1979; 29(13): 1077–1088.

Table 3.3 Sites and frequency of distant metastases	
Liver	38–60%
Abdominal lymph nodes	39%
Lung	38%
Peritoneum	28%
Ovary	18%
Adrenal glands	14%
Pleura	11%
Brain	8%
Bone	10%

Adapted from Kemeny N, Seiter K: Colon and rectal carcinoma. In: Handbook of Chemotherapy in Clinical Oncology. SCI Ltd. 1993; 589–594.

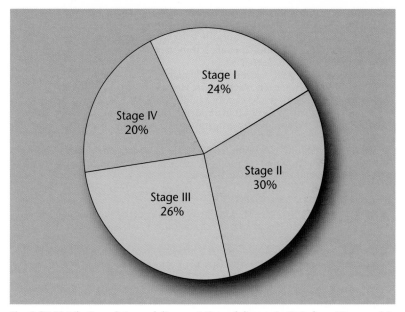

Fig. 3.36 Distribution of stage of disease at time of diagnosis. Data from Newman LA, Lee CT, Patel Parekh L, et al: Use of the National Cancer Data Base to develop clinical trials accrual targets that are appropriate for minority ethnicity patients: a report from the American College of Surgeons Oncology Group (ACOSOG) Special Population Committee. Cancer 2006; 106(1): 188–195.

REFERENCES

1. Jemal A, Siegel R, Ward E, et al: Cancer statistics, 2007. CA Cancer J Clin 2007; 57: 43–66.
2. Parkin DM, Bray F, Ferlay J, et al: Global cancer statistics, 2002. CA Cancer J Clin 2005; 55:74–108.
3. Lynch HT, de la Chapelle A: Hereditary colorectal cancer. N Engl J Med 2003; 348: 919–932.
4. Galiatsatos P, Foulkes WD: Familial adenomatous polyposis. Am J Gastroenterol 2006; 101: 385–398.
5. Lynch HT, Smyrk TC, Watson P, et al: Genetics, natural history, tumor spectrum, and pathology of hereditary nonpolyposis colorectal cancer: an updated review. Gastroenterology 1993; 104: 1535–1549.
6. Ekbom A, Helmick C, Zack M, et al: Ulcerative colitis and colorectal cancer. A population-based study. N Engl J Med 1990; 323: 1228–1233.
7. Krok KL, Lichtenstein GR: Colorectal cancer in inflammatory bowel disease. Curr Opin Gastroenterol 2004; 20: 43–48.
8. Jess T, Gamborg M, Matzen P, et al: Increased risk of intestinal cancer in Crohn's disease: a meta-analysis of population-based cohort studies. Am J

Gastroenterol 2005; 100: 2724–2729.

9. Larsson SC, Orsini N, Wolk A: Diabetes mellitus and risk of colorectal cancer: a meta-analysis. J Natl Cancer Inst 2005; 97: 1679–1687.

10. Ron E, Gridley G, Hrubec Z, et al: Acromegaly and gastrointestinal cancer. Cancer 1991; 68: 1673–1677.

11. Barzilay J, Heatley GJ, Cushing GW: Benign and malignant tumors in patients with acromegaly. Arch Intern Med 1991; 151: 1629–1632.

12. Willett WC: Nutrition and cancer. Salud Publica Mex 1997; 39: 298–309.

13. Norat T, Bingham S, Ferrari P, et al: Meat, fish, and colorectal cancer risk: the European Prospective Investigation into cancer and nutrition. J Natl Cancer Inst 2005; 97: 906–916.

14. Chan AT, Tranah GJ, Giovannucci EL, et al: Prospective study of N-acetyltransferase-2 genotypes, meat intake, smoking and risk of colorectal cancer. Int J Cancer 2005; 115: 648–652.

15. Chao A, Thun MJ, Connell CJ, et al: Meat consumption and risk of colorectal cancer. JAMA 2005; 293: 172–182.

16. Giovannucci E, Stampfer MJ, Colditz GA, et al: Folate, methionine, and alcohol intake and risk of colorectal adenoma. J Natl Cancer Inst 1993; 85: 875–884.

17. Kesse E, Boutron-Ruault MC, Norat T, et al: Dietary calcium, phosphorus, vitamin D, dairy products and the risk of colorectal adenoma and cancer among French women of the E3N-EPIC prospective study. Int J Cancer 2005; 117: 137–144.

18. McCullough ML, Robertson AS, Rodriguez C, et al: Calcium, vitamin D, dairy products, and risk of colorectal cancer in the Cancer Prevention Study II Nutrition Cohort (United States). Cancer Causes Control 2003; 14: 1–12.

19. Giovannucci E, Liu Y, Rimm EB, et al: Prospective study of predictors of vitamin D status and cancer incidence and mortality in men. J Natl Cancer Inst 2006; 98: 451–459.

20. Terry P, Giovannucci E, Michels KB, et al: Fruit, vegetables, dietary fiber, and risk of colorectal cancer. J Natl Cancer Inst 2001; 93: 525–533.

21. Flood A, Velie EM, Chaterjee N, et al: Fruit and vegetable intakes and the risk of colorectal cancer in the Breast Cancer Detection Demonstration Project follow-up cohort. Am J Clin Nutr 2002; 75: 936–943.

22. Lin J, Zhang SM, Cook NR, et al: Dietary intakes of fruit, vegetables, and fiber, and risk of colorectal cancer in a prospective cohort of women (United States). Cancer Causes Control 2005; 16: 225–233.

23. Park Y, Hunter DJ, Spiegelman D, et al: Dietary fiber intake and risk of colorectal cancer: a pooled analysis of prospective cohort studies. JAMA 2005; 294: 2849–2857.

24. Bingham SA, Norat T, Moskal A, et al: Is the association with fiber from foods in colorectal cancer confounded by folate intake? Cancer Epidemiol Biomarkers Prev 2005; 14: 1552–1556.

25. Fuchs CS, Giovannucci EL, Colditz GA, et al: Dietary fiber and the risk of colorectal cancer and adenoma in women. N Engl J Med 1999; 340: 169–176.

26. Giovannucci E, Ascherio A, Rimm EB, et al: Physical activity, obesity, and risk for colon cancer and adenoma in men. Ann Intern Med 1995; 122: 327–334.

27. Martinez ME, Giovannucci E, Spiegelman D, et al: Leisure-time physical activity, body size, and colon cancer in women. Nurses' Health Study

Research Group. J Natl Cancer Inst 1997; 89: 948–955.

28. Lee IM, Paffenbarger RS, Jr., Hsieh C: Physical activity and risk of developing colorectal cancer among college alumni. J Natl Cancer Inst 1991; 83: 1324–1329.

29. Calle EE, Rodriguez C, Walker-Thurmond K, et al: Overweight, obesity, and mortality from cancer in a prospectively studied cohort of U.S. adults. N Engl J Med 2003; 348: 1625–1638.

30. Slattery ML: Physical activity and colorectal cancer. Sports Med 2004; 34: 239–252.

31. Giovannucci E: Nutrition, insulin, insulin-like growth factors and cancer. Horm Metab Res 2003; 35: 694–704.

32. Kaaks R, Lukanova A: Energy balance and cancer: the role of insulin and insulin-like growth factor-I. Proc Nutr Soc 2001; 60: 91–106.

33. McKeown-Eyssen G: Epidemiology of colorectal cancer revisited: are serum triglycerides and/or plasma glucose associated with risk? Cancer Epidemiol Biomarkers Prev 1994; 3: 687–695.

34. Sturmer T, Glynn RJ, Lee IM, et al: Lifetime cigarette smoking and colorectal cancer incidence in the Physicians' Health Study I. J Natl Cancer Inst 2000; 92: 1178–1181.

35. Chao A, Thun MJ, Jacobs EJ, et al: Cigarette smoking and colorectal cancer mortality in the cancer prevention study II. J Natl Cancer Inst 2000; 92: 1888–1896.

36. Narisawa T, Sato M, Tani M, et al: Inhibition of development of methyl-nitrosourea-induced rat colon tumors by indomethacin treatment. Cancer Res 1981; 41: 1954–1957.

37. Reddy BS, Maruyama H, Kelloff G: Dose-related inhibition of colon carcinogenesis by dietary piroxicam, a nonsteroidal antiinflammatory drug, during different stages of rat colon tumor development. Cancer Res 1987; 47: 5340–5346.

38. Moorghen M, Ince P, Finney KJ, et al: A protective effect of sulindac against chemically-induced primary colonic tumours in mice. J Pathol 1988; 156: 341–347.

39. Kune GA, Kune S, Watson LF: Colorectal cancer risk, chronic illnesses, operations, and medications: case control results from the Melbourne Colorectal Cancer Study. Cancer Res 1988; 48: 4399–4404.

40. Thun MJ, Namboodiri MM, Heath CW, Jr.: Aspirin use and reduced risk of fatal colon cancer. N Engl J Med 1991; 325: 1593–1596.

41. Chan AT, Giovannucci EL, Meyerhardt JA, et al: Long-term use of aspirin and nonsteroidal anti-inflammatory drugs and risk of colorectal cancer. JAMA 2005; 294: 914–923.

42. Rigau J, Pique JM, Rubio E, et al: Effects of long-term sulindac therapy on colonic polyposis. Ann Intern Med 1991; 115: 952–954.

43. Labayle D, Fischer D, Vielh P, et al: Sulindac causes regression of rectal polyps in familial adenomatous polyposis. Gastroenterology 1991; 101: 635–639.

44. Giardiello FM, Hamilton SR, Krush AJ, et al: Treatment of colonic and rectal adenomas with sulindac in familial adenomatous polyposis. N Engl J Med 1993; 328: 1313–1316.

45. Baron JA, Cole BF, Sandler RS, et al: A randomized trial of aspirin to prevent colorectal adenomas. N Engl J Med 2003; 348: 891–899.

46. Sandler RS, Halabi S, Baron JA, et al: A randomized trial of aspirin to prevent colorectal adenomas in patients with previous colorectal cancer. N

Engl J Med 2003; 348: 883–890.

47. Jacobs EJ, Rodriguez C, Brady KA, et al: Cholesterol-lowering drugs and colorectal cancer incidence in a large United States cohort. J Natl Cancer Inst 2006; 98: 69–72.

48. Poynter JN, Gruber SB, Higgins PD, et al: Statins and the risk of colorectal cancer. N Engl J Med 2005; 352: 2184–2192.

49. Fearon ER, Vogelstein B: A genetic model for colorectal tumorigenesis. Cell 1990; 61: 759–767.

50. Greene F, Page D, Fleming I, et al: AJCC Cancer Staging Handbook (ed 6). New York, Springer, 2002.

51. Greene FL, Stewart AK, Norton HJ: A new TNM staging strategy for node-positive (stage III) colon cancer: an analysis of 50,042 patients. Ann Surg 2002; 236: 416–421; discussion 421.

Colorectal cancer therapy

4

Jeffrey Meyerhardt

Treatment for colorectal cancer (CRC) depends on stage of disease (see Table 4.1). The bases of the treatment algorithm are both the potential curability of the disease and likelihood of recurrence. The principal treatment modalities utilized are surgery, chemotherapy and radiation therapy.

Table 4.1 Treatment paradigms for colorectal cancer		
	Colon cancer	**Rectal cancer**
Stage I ($T_{1-2} N_0 M_0$)	Surgery	Surgery
Stage II ($T_{3-4} N_0 M_0$)	Surgery +/− Chemotherapy *	Chemotherapy/radiation (chemoradiation) followed by surgery followed by chemotherapy † or Surgery followed by chemoradiation and chemotherapy †
Stage III ($T_{any} N_{1-2} M_0$)	Surgery followed by chemotherapy	Chemoradiation followed by surgery followed by chemotherapy † or Surgery followed by chemoradiation and chemotherapy †
Stage IV ($T_{any} N_{any} M_1$)	Chemotherapy (consider palliative surgery) ††	Chemotherapy (consider palliative surgery)††

NOTE: For patients with rectal cancer who receive neoadjuvant chemoradiation, stage is defined by endoscopic ultrasound or pelvic magnetic resonance imaging.

* Chemotherapy for stage II colon cancer is controversial though certain high-risk features are considered when deciding on adjuvant therapy.

† Studies for stage II and III rectal cancer included use of both chemoradiation and chemotherapy though the benefit of chemotherapy in addition to that used with radiation has not been definitively proven.

†† Selected patients with limited Stage IV disease may be candidates for curative-intent surgery for metastases.

SURGERY

Surgery is considered the only curative therapy for CRCs. While other modalities, including chemotherapy and radiation, are critical components of many patients' treatment, a critical step in approaching patients is determining the suitability and timing of surgery. Eighty percent of patients will present without detectable metastases. For such patients with colon cancer, surgery is usually the first step in treatment. For patients with rectal cancer, preoperative staging with either pelvis magnetic resonance imaging (MRI) or endorectal ultrasound is required to determine whether the patient has clinically stage II or III disease; in most patients with stage II or III disease, neoadjuvant combined chemotherapy and radiation should be offered.[1] Alternatively, for patients with metastatic disease, removal of the primary tumour still remains an important consideration to palliate and prevent symptoms due to the colorectal lesion (including bleeding and obstruction).

SURGERY OF PRIMARY TUMOUR

The basic principles of surgery for CRC include *en bloc* resection to achieve a complete resection with negative margins, lymphadenectomy to the level of the origin of the primary feeding vessel and removal and examination of at least 12 regional lymph nodes.[2] The surgeon should explore the abdomen intraoperatively to rule out metastases to the peritoneum, distant lymph nodes or other visceral organs. For colon cancer, increasing evidence suggests that a laparoscopic colectomy can be an alternative to open colectomy without compromising long-term outcomes when performed by surgeons with experience in the technique (see Figures 4.1, 4.2 and 4.3).[3–5] For rectal cancer, a wide anatomical resection of the mesorectum with ideal bowel margins at least 2 cm distally and 5 cm proximally and clear radial margins is optimal (see Figure 3.4).[2] Concerns about achieving negative lateral and circumferential margins have been addressed by the wider acceptance of total mesorectal excision (TME) for rectal cancers. Conventional surgery violates the mesorectal circumference during blunt dissection, leaving residual mesorectum in the pelvis. TME is performed by a sharp and extensive resection of the mesorectum in an attempt to reduce the likelihood of a local recurrence and reduce potential surgical toxicities like impotence and urinary incontinence. Randomized trials of blunt dissection versus TME have not been reported, and increased operative times and risk of anastomotic leakages have tempered universal acceptance. Nonetheless, with the exception of low rectal cancers, TME appears to decrease the risk of involvement of the circumferential margin, which is strongly predictive of the risk of local recurrences.[6]

METASTATIC DISEASE

Twenty percent of patients diagnosed with CRC will have metastases at the time of initial presentation and another 25–50% of patients initially diagnosed with local or localized advanced disease will develop metastases. Of patients first discovered to have metastatic disease, 50% will appear to have disease limited to their liver, and at the time of death 20% appear to still have only liver metastases.[7] Increasingly, surgeons and

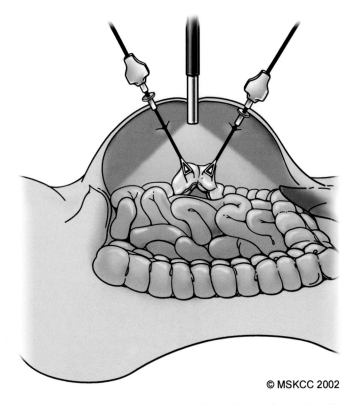

© MSKCC 2002

Fig. 4.1 Laparascopic colectomy is performed with the use of gas to insufflate the abdomen, video to visualize internally and trocars to perform all surgical manoeuvres. Reproduced with permission from Memorial Sloan Kettering Cancer Center.

medical oncologists have attempted to surgically cure patients with limited metastatic disease. Nonetheless, less than 10% of patients with metastatic disease are considered surgical candidates for metastatectomies. Positron emission tomography (PET) scans and MRI are helpful adjuncts to traditional computed tomography (CT) staging in determining appropriateness for surgical resection of liver metastases.

Historical series suggest that the cure rate from this highly selected group of patients that undergo liver metastases resections (see Figure 4.4) is up to 30%.[7] Various scoring systems have been developed to predict which patients would benefit from attempted surgery. Criteria that have consistently been accepted as portending an increased likelihood of extrahepatic disease or disease recurrence include lymph node positive primary tumour, synchronous primary and metastases, recurrence of disease less than 12 months after primary removal, multiple liver metastases or multiple lobar disease, preoperative or postoperative serum carcinoembryonic antigen (CEA) elevation, or any lesion greater than 5 cm

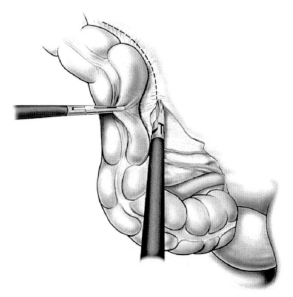

Fig. 4.2 The dissection of the lateral attachments of the sigmoid and left colon using laparoscopic instruments. Reproduced with permission from Weiser MR, Milsom JW: Laparoscopic total mesorectal excision with autonomic nerve preservation. Semin Surg Oncol 2000; 19(4): 396–403.

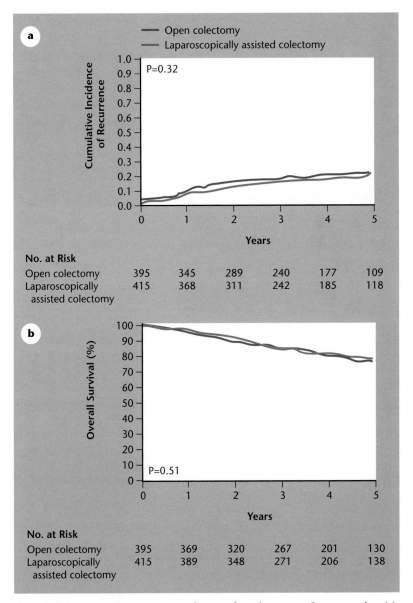

Fig. 4.3 3 Laparascopic versus open colectomy for colon cancer. Recurrence-free (**a**) and overall survival (**b**) Kaplan-Meier curves for all stage (stage I–III) patients. Reproduced with permission from The Clinical Outcomes of Surgical Therapy Study Group: A comparison of laparoscopically assisted and open colectomy for colon cancer. N Engl J Med 2004; 350: 2050–2059. © Massachusetts Medical Society.

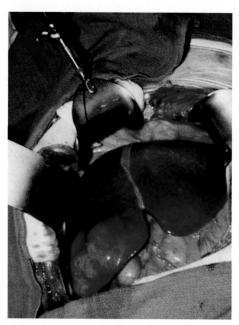

Fig. 4.4 Liver tumour exposed in segment 5 of the right liver lobe at the time of resection. (Courtesy of Dr Kenneth Tanabe, Massachusetts General Hospital, Boston, MA.)

in size.[8,9] While more aggressive approaches have been suggested including allowing multilobar disease, unlimited size or number of metastases, extrahepatic disease and intraoperative ablation for difficult surgical margins,[7] prospective data should be obtained to evaluate whether such patients truly benefit from such an aggressive approach. Further, with the availability of more active agents against metastatic disease, there is hope that neoadjuvant therapy with combination regimens will increase the number of patients where such resections should be considered.[10] In a proof-of-principle retrospective study, evaluating a variant schedule of fluorouracil, leucovorin and oxaliplatin, investigators demonstrated that first-line cytotoxic chemotherapy had downsized a significant fraction of unresectable disease to operability.[11] Specifically, following the treatment of 151 patients with liver-only, previously inoperable metastatic disease, 77 were subsequently resected with curative intent. Median overall survival in this group was 48 months against 15.5 months in the non-operated patients. A recent analysis of all published trials and retrospective studies that had reported tumour response and resection rates of initially unresectable hepatic lesions highlighted how effective this approach can be in advanced CRC. For patients with inoperable metastases confined to the liver (selected patients), resection rates after first-line chemotherapy with a range of regimens were 24–54%; for all patients with advanced disease (unselected patients), the rate was 1–26%. A highly significant correlation between tumour response and resection rate was seen for both selected and unselected patients, suggesting that regimens that produce the highest response rates are likely to be those that allow the highest hepatic resection rates.[12] One factor that should be considered in such evaluations is that a partial response to treatment is often sufficient and preferable for the facilitation of potentially curative liver resection. Nonetheless, long-term data on these patients remain to be reported and will be necessary to evaluate whether more aggressive downstaging actually alters the cure rate of this disease.

CHEMOTHERAPY

Chemotherapy is an important component of the treatment of patients with metastatic disease as well as many patients with surgically resected tumours (see Table 4.2). The backbone of CRC treatment for the past three decades has been the fluorinated pyrimidine 5-fluorouracil (5-FU). Recently, multiple new agents have been added to the treatment armamentarium for CRC. In addition to intravenous fluorouracil, oral derivations of fluorouracil include capecitabine and uracil plus tegafur (UFT). Two other traditional cytotoxic therapies that have definitive activity against CRC include irinotecan and oxaliplatin. Finally, more specific targeted therapies against the vascular endothelial growth factor (bevacizumab) and epidermal growth factor receptor (EGFR; cetuximab and panitumumab) are having an expanding role against CRC.

FLUOROPYRIMIDINES

Fluorouracil is thought to act primarily by inhibiting thymidylate synthase, the rate-limiting enzyme for pyrimidine nucleotide synthesis. It is usually administered with leucovorin, a reduced folate which stabilizes the binding of fluorouracil to thymidylate synthase, thereby enhancing the inhibition of DNA synthesis (see Figure 4.5).[13] In patients with advanced CRC, 5-FU and leucovorin provides a 20% response rate and prolongs median survival from approximately 6 months (without treatment) to about 11 months.[14–17]

The establishment of 5-FU as adjuvant therapy was based on two trials completed in the late 1980s. The North Central Cancer Treatment Group (NCCTG) randomized 401 patients with stage II or III colon cancer to

Table 4.2 Common chemotherapy regimens for colorectal cancer

Regimen	Chemotherapy dosing	Schedule
Fluoropyrimidines		
Roswell Park	5-FU 500 mg/m^2 bolus + LV 500 mg/m^2	Weekly for 6 of 8 weeks
Mayo Clinic	5-FU 425 mg/m^2 bolus days 1–5 LV 20 mg/m^2 bolus days 1–5	Every 4–5 weeks
LV5FU2	Intravenous 5-FU 400 mg/m^2 bolus on days 1,2 600 mg/m^2 IVCI over 22 hours on days 1,2 + LV 200 mg/m^2 on days 1,2	Every 2 weeks
Arbeitsgemeinschaft Internische Onkologie (AIO)	5-FU 2000 mg/m^2 IVCI x 24 hours LV 500 mg/m^2	Weekly for 6 of 8 weeks
Capecitabine	1250 mg/m^2 orally twice per day on days 1–14	Every 3 weeks
Irinotecan		
IFL	5-FU 125 mg/m^2 on day 1 LV 20 mg/m^2 on day 1 Irinotecan 125 mg/m^2 on day 1	Weekly for 4 of 6 weeks. Users often modify to 2 of 3 weeks
Douillard	5-FU 400 mg/m^2 bolus + 600 mg/m^2 IVCI over 22 hours days 1,2 LV 200 mg/m^2 on days 1,2 Irinotecan 180 mg/m^2 on day 1	Every 2 weeks
FOLFIRI	5-FU 400 mg/m^2 bolus on day 1 + 2400–3000 mg/m^2 IVCI over 46 hours on days 1,2 LV 200 mg/m^2 on day 1 Irinotecan 180 mg/m^2 on day 1	Every 2 weeks

observation, adjuvant treatment with levamisole or adjuvant treatment with levamisole and fluorouracil.[18] After a median follow-up of 8 years, patients treated with levamisole and fluorouracil had a 31% reduction in recurrence, and a small improvement in overall survival was seen in patients with stage III disease (see Figure 4.6). No benefit was observed in patients who received levamisole alone. These results were confirmed in a larger Intergroup trial of nearly 1300 patients with stage II and III

Table 4.2 *Continued* **Common chemotherapy regimens for colorectal cancer**

Regimen	Chemotherapy dosing	Schedule
Oxaliplatin		
FOLFOX4	5-FU 400 mg/m^2 bolus + 600 mg/m^2 IVCI over 22 hours days 1,2 LV 200 mg/m^2 on days 1,2 Oxaliplatin 85 mg/m^2 on day 1	Every 2 weeks
FOLFOX6	5-FU 400 mg/m^2 bolus on day 1 + 2400–3000 mg/m^2 IVCI over 46 hours on days 1,2 LV 200 mg/m^2 on day 1 Oxaliplatin 100 mg/m^2 on day 1	Every 2 weeks
Modified FOLFOX6	5-FU 400 mg/m^2 bolus on day 1 + 2400–3000 mg/m^2 IVCI over 46 hours on days 1,2 LV 200 mg/m^2 on day 1 Oxaliplatin 85 mg/m^2 on day 1	Every 2 weeks
Bevacizumab		
Intravenous 5-FU containing regimens	Bevacizumab 5 mg/kg or 10 mg/kg on day 1 in addition to cytotoxic chemotherapies	Every 2 weeks
Cetuximab		
Cetuximab single agent	Cetuximab 400 mg/m^2 loading dose and then 250 mg/m^2 subsequently	Weekly
Cetuximab + irinotecan	Cetuximab 400 mg/m^2 loading dose and then 250 mg/m^2 subsequently weekly irinotecan 125 mg/m^2 weekly x 4 then 2 weeks off or irinotecan 180 mg/m^2 every other week or irinotecan 350 mg/m^2 every third week	Weekly cetuximab Varied for irinotecan
Panitumumab		
Panitumumab single agent	Panitumumab 6 mg/kg	Every 2 weeks

5-FU, 5-fluorouracil; LV, leucovorin; IVCI, intravenous continuous infusion

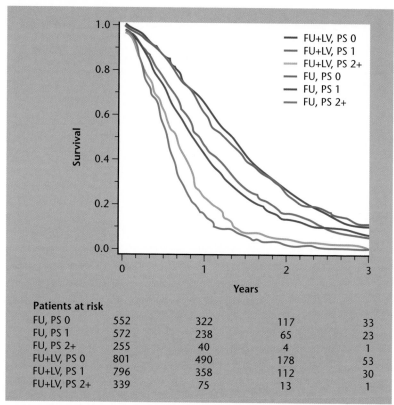

Fig. 4.5 Survival curves with 5-fluorouracil (FU) or 5-fluorouracil with leucovorin (LV) in patients with metastatic colorectal cancer. Leucovorin leads to a modest improvement in survival. Performance status is also predictive of survival. Performance status: PS 0 = fully active; PS 1 = restricted in physically strenuous activity but ambulatory and able to carry out light work; PS 2 = ambulatory and capable of all self-care but unable to carry out any work activities, up and about more than 50% of waking hours. Reproduced from Thirion P, Michiels S, Pignon JP, et al: Modulation of fluorouracil by leucovorin in patients with advanced colorectal cancer: an updated meta-analysis. J Clin Oncol 2004; 22: 3766–3775. Reprinted with permission from the American Society of Clinical Oncology.

colon cancer. In patients with stage III disease, treatment with adjuvant fluorouracil and levamisole reduced the risk of recurrence by 41% and the risk of death by 33% compared with surgery alone.[19] These risk reductions were preserved with longer follow-up of 6.5 years.[20] In contrast, no benefit was seen in patients with stage II disease. Subsequent trials confirmed similar benefits of adjuvant therapy as well as substituting leucovorin for levamisole as a modulator of fluorouracil activity.[21–23] In

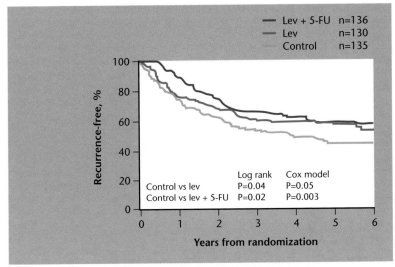

Fig. 4.6 Recurrence-free survival benefit of adjuvant 5-fluorouracil (5-FU) and levamisole (Lev) in stage II/III colon cancer. Kaplan-Meier curve comparing surgery only with levamisole adjuvant therapy to combined 5-fluorouracil and levamisole adjuvant therapy. Reproduced from Laurie JA, Moertel CG, Fleming TR, et al: Surgical adjuvant therapy of large-bowel carcinoma: an evaluation of levamisole and the combination of levamisole and fluorouracil. The North Central Cancer Treatment Group and the Mayo Clinic. J Clin Oncol 1989; 7: 1447–1456. Reprinted with permission from the American Society of Clinical Oncology.

1990, a National Cancer Institute consensus conference recommended fluorouracil-based adjuvant therapy as the standard of care for patients with resected stage III colon cancer.[24]

The major side effects associated with fluorouracil are dependent upon the method of administration. When the drug is given using a "loading" schedule of bolus treatments on 5 consecutive days every 4–5 weeks, neutropenia and stomatitis are the most common toxicities. In contrast, diarrhoea is more frequent with weekly bolus doses. Regimens involving intravenous infusions of fluorouracil (administered as a continuous infusion with a portable infusion pump) are associated with less haematological and gastrointestinal toxicity, but palmar-plantar erythrodysaesthesia ("hand–foot" syndrome) is more common.[25–27] While constant intravenous infusion regimens were previously perceived as being more expensive and less convenient than bolus regimens, recent analyses suggest that differences in cost and quality of life between the bolus and prolonged infusion schedules are marginal.[28,29] Furthermore, continuous infusion appears to be moderately more effective than a rapid bolus approach.[30]

Initial attempts to administer fluorouracil orally were disappointing. A double-blind, placebo-controlled, randomized study showed intravenous fluorouracil to be more effective than an oral form.[31] Pharmacokinetic plasma assays suggested that this superiority was due to the erratic intestinal absorption of oral fluorouracil, possibly reflecting variable mucosal concentrations of dihydropyrimidine dehydrogenase, a major catabolic enzyme of the drug. Strategies developed to overcome this problem include the administration of prodrugs of fluorouracil that are absorbed intact and are metabolically activated following intestinal absorption[32] or the co-administration of oral fluorouracil with drugs that inhibit the action of dihydropyrimidine dehydrogenase.[33–35]

Capecitabine is a prodrug that undergoes a three-step enzymatic conversion to fluorouracil (see Figures 4.7 and 4.8).[32] The side effect profile

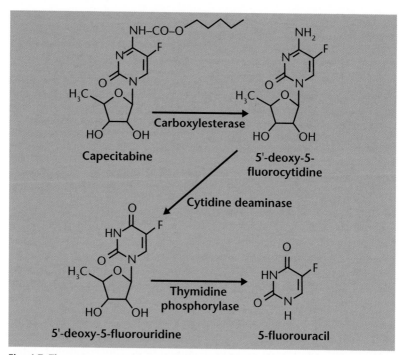

Fig. 4.7 Three-step enzymatic process of conversion of capecitabine to 5-fluorouracil (5-FU). Capecitabine is absorbed from the gastrointestinal tract and processed in the liver to 5'-deoxy-5-fluorocytidine (5'-DFCR). Cytidine deaminase, an enzyme found in most tissues, including tumours, subsequently converts 5'-DFCR to 5'-deoxy-5-fluorouridine (5'-DFUR). The enzyme thymidine phosphorylase then hydrolyzes 5'-DFUR to the active drug 5-FU. Though many tissues normally express thymidine phosphorylase, it is markedly upregulated in certain tumours.

of capecitabine is similar to that observed with protracted infusions of 5-FU. Hand–foot syndrome is a prominent toxicity, and other adverse reactions include diarrhoea, nausea, vomiting and bone marrow suppression.[36–38] Two randomized clinical trials comparing capecitabine to the monthly schedule of fluorouracil and leucovorin[36,37] reported that patients treated with capecitabine experienced a modest improvement in objective response (19–25% as compared with 15%) while median overall survival (12–13 months) was similar with either regimen. Patients receiving intravenous fluorouracil with the loading regimen were more likely to develop mouth sores and bone marrow suppression, while patients allocated to receive capecitabine had an increased incidence of hand–foot syndrome.

In the adjuvant setting, capecitabine has also demonstrated comparable efficacy to the loading regimen of monthly bolus fluorouracil and leucovorin in patients with stage III colon cancer.[39] The Xeloda in Adjuvant Colon Cancer Therapy (X-ACT) trial randomized 1,987 patients with stage III colon cancer to capecitabine or a loading schedule of fluorouracil and leucovorin for 24 weeks.[39] With median follow-up of 3.8 years, disease-free survival was statistically equivalent in the two arms (64% vs. 61%). In addition, 3-year overall survival was similar in the two arms (81% capecitabine vs. 78% fluorouracil and leucovorin).

An example of an oral fluorouracil combination that inhibits dihydropyrimidine dehydrogenase is UFT, which has been approved by regulatory agencies outside the US. Tegafur, a prodrug of fluorouracil, is combined with a competitive blocker of dihydropyrimidine dehydrogenase (uracil) to improve the absorption and bioavailability of tegafur.[34] The drug is usually administered with oral leucovorin. In two randomized studies for metastatic disease, this therapy resulted in a similar response rate and median overall survival as compared with parenteral fluorouracil and leucovorin.[40,41] In addition, UFT and leucovorin appear to be equivalent to intravenous fluorouracil and leucovorin as adjuvant therapy for patients with stage II and III colon cancer.[42]

Fluoropyrimidines remain an important component of the treatment of metastatic CRC as well as in adjuvant therapy. Given the recent addition of other agents to the choices of therapy, patients rarely receive

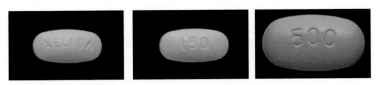

Fig. 4.8 Capecitabine tablets. Images courtesy of Roche.

fluoropyrimidines only for metastatic disease. However, patients with metastatic disease and a poor performance status or those who cannot tolerate more aggressive regimens should still be considered candidates for this treatment. As adjuvant therapy, combination regimens are increasingly utilized for stage III and some stage II patients. Nonetheless, intravenous 5-FU and leucovorin or capecitabine remain established therapies to offer patients.

IRINOTECAN

Irinotecan, also known as CPT-11, is a semisynthetic derivative of the natural alkaloid camptothecin, which exerts its cytotoxic effect through its interaction with the enzyme topoisomerase I (see Figure 4.9).[43] This enzyme is involved in DNA uncoiling for replication and transcription, and it causes single-stranded DNA breaks. Such breaks are normally transient and repaired; however, camptothecins stabilize these breaks, leading to DNA fragmentation and cell death through collision with the replication fork.

Irinotecan is a prodrug that is hydrolysed to its active metabolite, SN-38, by hepatic carboxylesterases. SN-38 is detoxified to an inactive glucuronidated form (SN-38G) by uridine diphosphate glucuronosyltransferase isoform 1A1 (UGT1A1) and is excreted in the urine and bile.[44] Additionally, several other inactive metabolites of irinotecan are formed through oxidative metabolism by the P450 enzymes, CYP3A4 and CYP3A5.[45]

The toxicities of irinotecan include diarrhoea, bone marrow suppression, nausea, vomiting and alopecia. Polymorphisms of uridine diphosphate glucuronosyltransferase isoform 1A1 appear to correlate with the severity of gastrointestinal toxicities and bone marrow suppression.[46–48]

Two randomized trials established the efficacy of single-agent irinotecan in second-line treatment of patients with metastatic CRC who progressed on prior fluorouracil-based therapy.[49,50] Median overall survival was extended by 2–3 months with a similar or improved quality of life in the irinotecan groups versus either best supportive care or continuous infusion fluorouracil. Two subsequent trials demonstrated superior efficacy of irinotecan combined with either infusional or bolus fluorouracil and leucovorin when compared with fluorouracil and leucovorin alone as first-line therapy in metastatic disease (see Figure 4.10).[51–52] Median overall survival was again improved by 2–3 months with a doubling of objective response rate from approximately 20% to 40%. A recent randomized study demonstrated that the infusional regimen of 5-FU,

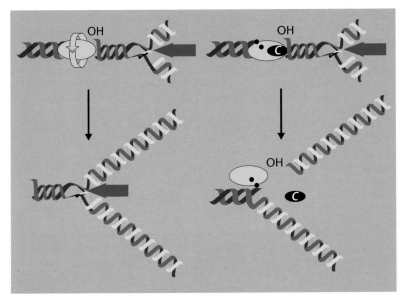

Fig. 4.9 Irinotecan mechanism of action. Topoisomerase I causes a very transient nick in the DNA to allow the release of torsion of the double strand as DNA replicates; the DNA break is re-ligated quickly. Irinotecan (C) binds to the topoisomerase-DNA complex and prevents re-ligation and release of topoisomerase, leading to double-strand breaks. Reproduced with permission from Rivory LP: New drugs for colorectal cancer – mechanism of action. Aust Prescr 2002; 25: 108–110.

leucovorin and irinotecan (FOLFIRI) has superior efficacy and less toxicity compared with the bolus regimen (IFL).[53]

Three randomized trials have tested the potential benefit of adding irinotecan with either bolus or infusional fluorouracil and leucovorin as adjuvant therapy.[53–55] A North American trial of over 1,200 patients with resected stage III colon cancer failed to show any benefit of adding irinotecan to a weekly schedule of fluorouracil and leucovorin.[53] The Pan European Trials in Adjuvant Colon Cancer (PETACC)-3 trial randomized over 3,000 patients with resected stage II and III colon cancer to receive infusional fluorouracil and leucovorin with or without irinotecan.[54] An initial presentation of the data suggests that irinotecan did not improve disease-free survival or overall survival compared with fluorouracil and leucovorin alone. However, longer follow-up is needed to fully evaluate this trial as well as consideration that the definition of the primary end-point, disease-free survival, included new primary cancers of any type, an event not included in disease-free survival in other comparable trials

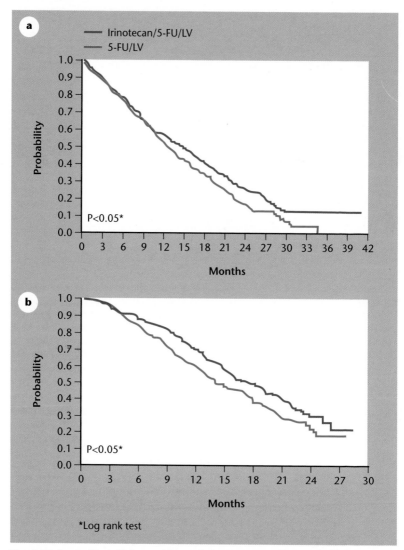

Fig. 4.10 Survival benefit from addition of irinotecan to 5-fluorouracil (5-FU) and leucovorin (LV) as initial therapy in patients with metastatic colorectal cancer. North America study (**a**) with bolus regimen and European study (**b**) with infusional regimen. (**a**) Data from Saltz LB, Cox JV, Blanke C, et al: Irinotecan plus fluorouracil and leucovorin for metastatic colorectal cancer. Irinotecan Study Group. N Engl J Med 2000; 343: 905–914. (**b**) Data from Douillard JY, Cunningham D, Roth AD, et al: Irinotecan combined with fluorouracil compared with fluorouracil alone as first-line treatment for metastatic colorectal cancer: a multicentre randomised trial. Lancet 2000; 355: 1041–1047.

(which usually define disease-free survival as time from enrollment until disease recurrence, new primary CRC or death). Nonetheless, a smaller European trial with a similar trial design to PETACC-3, though limited to high-risk stage III colon cancer (four or more positive lymph nodes or 1–3 positive lymph nodes with colonic obstruction or perforation), showed a worse, though not statistically different, 3-year disease-free survival in patients in the irinotecan-containing arm (51% vs. 60%).[55] Given these three trials and the increased toxicity of irinotecan when administered with fluorouracil and leucovorin, irinotecan currently cannot be recommended in the adjuvant setting for colon cancer.

OXALIPLATIN

Oxaliplatin is a third-generation platinum derivative that forms bulky DNA adducts and induces cellular apoptosis (see Figure 4.11).[56] Despite the ineffectiveness of other platinum drugs (such as cisplatin and carboplatin) in

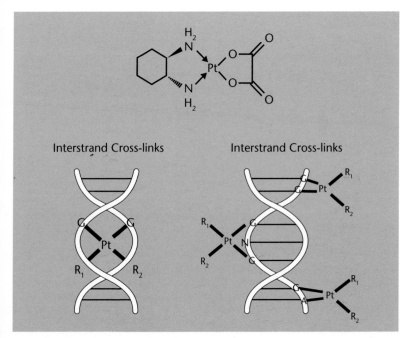

Fig. 4.11 Oxaliplatin and mechanism of action. Oxaliplatin forms inter- and intrastrand platinum-DNA adducts and cross-links, which inhibit DNA replication and transcription.

the treatment of CRC, preclinical data utilizing human cell lines suggested that oxaliplatin held promise in treating this disease.[57] Furthermore, oxaliplatin and fluorouracil were shown to be highly synergistic, not only in preclinical models,[58] but also in subsequent clinical trials.[59] A potential mechanism for this synergy is the downregulation of thymidylate synthase by oxaliplatin, thereby potentiating the efficacy of fluorouracil.[60]

The toxicity profile of oxaliplatin differs from that of cisplatin and carboplatin. Renal dysfunction, alopecia and ototoxicity are uncommon, but neuropathy is more frequent.[61] Two types of neuropathies have been described. Most patients experience transient dysaesthesias, manifested as numbness or tingling of the distal extremities, oral or perioral regions, which are exacerbated by exposure to cold temperatures. After months of therapy, patients can experience a cumulative, dose-dependent sensory neuropathy in which persistent peripheral dysaesthesias and paraesthesias remain between cycles of therapy, usually diminishing following cessation of treatment (see Figure 4.12).[62]

Although oxaliplatin as a single agent has limited efficacy when administered as initial[63–65] or second-line treatment[66] for patients with

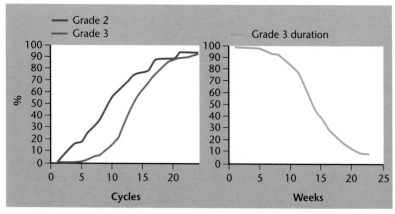

Fig. 4.12 Oxaliplatin neurotoxicity. Time frame for development of grade 2 (paraesthesias/dysaesthesias interfering with function, but not activities of daily living) and grade 3 (paraesthesias/dysaesthesias with pain or with functional impairment that also interfere with activities of daily living) neurotoxicity by number of cycles and recovery of grade 3 neurotoxicity after discontinuation of oxaliplatin. Reproduced from de Gramont A, Figer A, Seymour M, et al: Leucovorin and fluorouracil with or without oxaliplatin as first-line treatment in advanced colorectal cancer. J Clin Oncol 2000; 18: 2938–2947. Reprinted with permission from the American Society of Clinical Oncology.

metastatic CRC, significant benefit has been shown when the drug is combined with bolus fluorouracil and leucovorin followed by a 48-hour infusion of fluorouracil in a treatment regimen known as "FOL-FOX".[11,59,62,67] Efficacy of oxaliplatin in first-line treatment of metastatic CRC was demonstrated initially by two phase III trials that randomized patients to infusional fluorouracil and leucovorin with or without oxaliplatin.[11,62] Both studies showed a significant increase in the response rate and disease-free survival for patients in the oxaliplatin-containing arm, with a trend toward improved overall survival. A significant survival benefit for oxaliplatin, fluorouracil and leucovorin (FOL-FOX) was demonstrated in a North American multicentre trial (N9741) that randomized 795 patients with newly diagnosed metastatic CRC to receive FOLFOX, IFL or a combination of irinotecan and oxaliplatin (IROX). Overall survival favoured FOLFOX when compared with either IFL or IROX (19.5 months, 15.0 months and 17.4 months, respectively). Further studies have confirmed the efficacy of oxaliplatin in combination with fluorouracil and leucovorin as first-line and second-line treatment of metastatic CRC.[59,68]

Oxaliplatin has been shown to be beneficial as adjuvant therapy for patients with resected colon cancer. In the Multicenter International Study of Oxaliplatin/Fluorouracil/Leucovorin in the Adjuvant Treatment of Colon Cancer (MOSAIC) study, 2,246 patients with stage II (40%) and stage III (60%) colon cancer were randomized to receive the infusional fluorouracil regimen with or without oxaliplatin (see Figure 4.13).[69] The 4-year disease-free survival in patients with stage III disease was statistically superior in those patients who received oxaliplatin (70% vs. 61%).[70] Although a statistically significant benefit was not seen in those patients with stage II disease, a 5.4% absolute improvement in disease-free survival was noted in patients with "high-risk" stage II disease, defined as the presence of T4 tumour stage, bowel obstruction, tumour perforation, poorly differentiated histology, venous invasion or less than 10 examined lymph nodes. After 4 years of follow-up, the statistically significant improvement in overall survival has not been confirmed. In a concurrent effort, a cooperative group trial in the US (NSABP-C07) also found a statistically significant benefit in disease-free survival from oxaliplatin being added a weekly regimen of 5-FU and leucovorin.[42]

In addition to an improvement in disease-free survival, treatment-related toxicities are a consideration in the oxaliplatin adjuvant trials. In the MOSAIC trial, grade 3 or 4 neutropenia was more common in patients receiving FOLFOX (41% vs. 5%), although neutropenia complicated by fever or infection was relatively uncommon in both groups (2% vs. 0.2%).

Grade 3 neuropathy, defined as severe objective sensory loss or neuropathy that interfered with function, was also significantly more common in patients treated with FOLFOX (12.4% versus 0.2%), and persisted in a subset of patients (1.1%) 1 year after cessation of chemotherapy. Rates of diarrhoea, nausea and vomiting were also significantly higher in patients receiving oxaliplatin. Similarly, patients receiving oxaliplatin on NSABP-C07 also experienced higher rates of neurotoxicity that interfered with normal functioning (8% vs. 1%). In these patients, 0.5% had persistent grade 3 neurotoxicity 1 year after completing treatment.

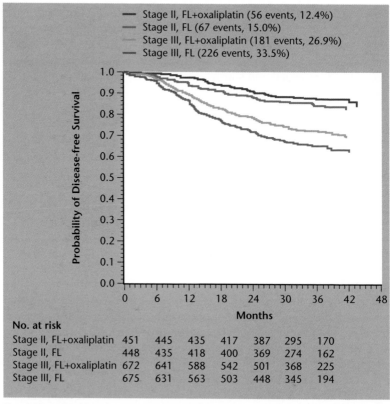

Fig. 4.13 MOSAIC trial results. The benefit of adding oxaliplatin to 5-fluorouracil and leucovorin (FL) in patients with stage II and III colon cancer. Reproduced with permission from Andre T, Boni C, Mounedji-Boudiaf L, et al: Oxaliplatin, fluorouracil, and leucovorin as adjuvant treatment for colon cancer. N Engl J Med 2004; 350: 2343–2351. © Massachusetts Medical Society.

EPIDERMAL GROWTH FACTOR RECEPTOR INHIBITORS

EGFR is a transmembrane glycoprotein that activates signalling pathways affecting cellular growth, differentiation, proliferation and programmed cell death.[71] It is expressed in malignancies of multiple tissues, including those of the colon, lung, breast, head and neck.[72] In CRC, EGFR expression has been demonstrated in up to 80% of tumours,[73,74] and tumours that express EGFR carry a poorer prognosis.[75] Antibodies directed against the extracellular domain of EGFR and small molecular inhibitors of the intracellular tyrosine kinase domain have been developed to inhibit the function of EGFR. Thus far, only the anti-EGFR monoclonal antibodies cetuximab and panitumumab have definitively demonstrated efficacy in CRC, although research is ongoing.[76–78]

In preclinical studies, antitumour activity was noted for cetuximab alone and in combination with chemotherapy in colon cancer cell lines.[79] In addition, synergistic antitumour activity was observed with the combination of the cetuximab and irinotecan in tumour cells sensitive to and resistant to irinotecan, suggesting that EGFR inhibition may overcome cellular resistance to irinotecan.[79] Due to these preclinical observations, clinical trials of cetuximab were initiated in CRC.

An initial phase II study involving 121 patients with advanced CRC enrolled patients whose tumours expressed EGFR and were refractory to irinotecan.[80] In this population, the combination of cetuximab and irinotecan resulted in a response rate of 19%. To determine whether this antineoplastic effect was due to synergy between the two drugs or to independent activity of cetuximab, 57 similar patients were treated with cetuximab alone, resulting in a 9% response rate (see Figure 4.14).[81] Similar response rates were noted in a larger, randomized phase II trial, in

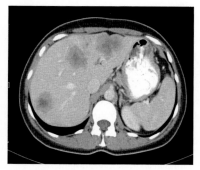 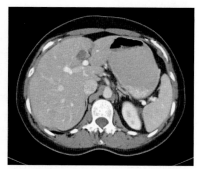

Fig. 4.14 Response to cetuximab (monotherapy) at 28 weeks. Left: before treatment. Right: after treatment.

which 329 patients with irinotecan-refractory, metastatic CRC received either cetuximab alone or cetuximab and irinotecan (see Figure 4.15).[82]

Investigations are ongoing to evaluate a role for cetuximab in adjuvant therapy of colon cancer. In two separate trials in North America and Europe, investigators are enrolling over 2,000 patients with resected stage III colon cancer to receive either FOLFOX or FOLFOX with cetuximab. These two parallel trials should provide data on the efficacy of cetuximab in the adjuvant setting.

The most common side effects of cetuximab are dermatological, including an acne-like rash, xerosis and fissures of the skin (see Figure 4.16).[82,83] While some degree of acneiform rash occurs in most patients, severe eruptions resulting in significant pain or infectious sequelae are less common.

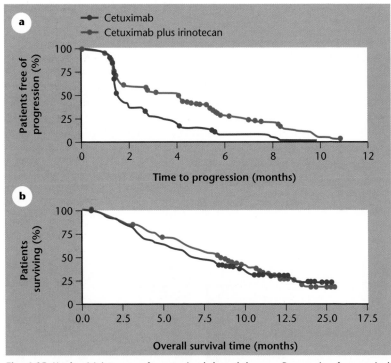

Fig. 4.15 Kaplan-Meier curves for cetuximab-based therapy. Progression-free survival (a) and overall survival (b) for cetuximab or cetuximab plus irinotecan in patients with metastatic colorectal cancer who previously progressed on irinotecan-based therapy. Reproduced with permission from Cunningham D, Humblet Y, Siena S, et al: Cetuximab monotherapy and cetuximab plus irinotecan in irinotecan-refractory metastatic colorectal cancer. N Engl J Med 2004; 351: 337–345. © Massachusetts Medical Society.

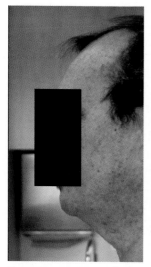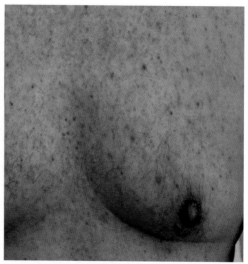

Fig. 4.16 Acneiform rash associated with cetuximab therapy.

Interestingly, the presence and severity of the cetuximab-induced rash, and not the level of EGFR expression, appears to correlate with the likelihood of tumour response.[82] In addition to dermatological toxicities, rare severe hypersensitivity infusional reactions can occur with cetuximab.

Panitumumab is a humanized monoclonal antibody to EGFR that has shown similar single-agent activity to cetuximab in metastatic CRC. In a phase II trial, 9% of patients whose cancer had progressed on fluorouracil and either irinotecan or oxaliplatin had a partial response to panitumumab, with a median progression-free survival of 3 months.[84] A phase III trial comparing panitumumab to best supportive care in patients with previously treated metastatic CRC found a statistically significant improvement in progression-free survival with panitumamab.[85]

ANGIOGENESIS INHIBITORS

Since tumours must induce the formation of blood vessels to allow continued growth, the inhibition of angiogenesis has been explored as a strategy to control the proliferation and spread of cancer cells.[86] At the current time, the most successful anti-angiogenic therapy has focused on inhibiting vascular endothelial growth factor (VEGF), a soluble protein that stimulates blood vessel proliferation.[87] Bevacizumab is a humanized monoclonal antibody directed against VEGF that has been examined in combination with chemotherapy in patients with advanced CRC.[88–90] In a randomized, phase III trial of previously untreated patients with metastatic disease, 815 patients were randomized to receive IFL with either bevacizumab or placebo (see Figure 4.17).[90] The addition of bevacizumab led to a statistically significant improvement in response rate (45% vs. 35%) and a 4.7 month prolongation in median overall survival (20.3 months vs. 15.6 months). In patients with metastatic CRC previously treated with fluorouracil and irinotecan, the combination of FOLFOX and bevacizumab has also demonstrated a statistically significant improvement in progression-free survival and overall survival when compared with FOLFOX alone.[91] The safety and efficacy of bevacizumab with first-line FOLFOX was confirmed by the TREE-2 study.[92]

Bevacizumab is relatively well tolerated, with reversible hypertension and proteinuria as two of the most common adverse events attributable to bevacizumab. Nonetheless, there are rare, yet serious side effects that have been observed consistently across CRC trials with bevacizumab, including a 1–2% risk of bowel perforation, 3% risk of serious bleeding events, and 2–3% risk of arterial embolic events.

The role of bevacizumab in adjuvant therapy for colon cancer is being studied in multiple randomized trials in the US and Europe. In addition to comparisons of disease-free survival, these trials will provide a critical examination of the rare but serious toxicities of bevacizumab in a curative-intent population (including bowel perforation and thromboembolic events). Until these trials are reported, data are not available to support the incorporation of bevacizumab into adjuvant therapy for colon cancer.

OPTIMAL ORDER OF THERAPY

The development of irinotecan, oxaliplatin, cetuximab and bevacizumab as treatment for CRC has been relatively rapid over the past decade. Though such choices in agents allow patients to have options for treatment if their tumour develops resistance or they do not tolerate a particular treatment, the rapid introduction into clinical practice has led to confusion as to the optimal order of therapy. Analyses from clinical trials suggest exposure to more agents at some time over the course of a patient's disease improves overall survival.[93]

Combination regimens should be considered for most chemo-naïve patients. Multiple randomized trials have compared irinotecan, fluorouracil and leucovorin regimens with oxaliplatin, fluorouracil and leucovorin combinations as initial treatment of metastatic CRC. In a multicentre trial conducted in North America, 795 patients were randomized

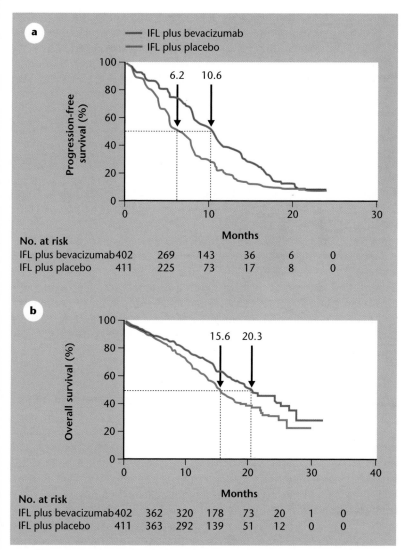

Fig. 4.17 Benefit of bevacizumab with chemotherapy as first-line therapy for metastatic colorectal cancer. Progression-free survival (**a**) and overall survival (**b**) on bevacizumab with a regimen of irinotecan, 5-fluorouracil and leucovorin (IFL). Reproduced with permission from Hurwitz H, Fehrenbacher L, Novotny W, et al: Bevacizumab plus irinotecan, fluorouracil, and leucovorin for metastatic colorectal cancer. N Engl J Med 2004; 350: 2335–2342. © Massachusetts Medical Society.

to receive either infusional 5-FU, leucovorin and oxaliplatin (FOLFOX) or weekly bolus irinotecan, 5-FU and leucovorin (IFL) or a combination of irinotecan with oxaliplatin (IROX).[94] The patients treated with FOLFOX experienced a superior response rate, time to disease progression and overall survival time when compared with either IFL or IROX (see Figure 4.18). However, this apparent superiority of FOLFOX may have been influenced by an imbalanced availability of second-line agents at the time the study was conducted, in that 60% of the patients initially treated with FOLFOX subsequently received irinotecan while only 24% on the IFL arm were then given oxaliplatin. Additionally, the IFL regimen utilizes a bolus fluorouracil schedule that may be inferior to the 2-day infusion of fluorouracil included in FOLFOX.[30] Nonetheless, these data support the option of oxaliplatin-based therapy as a first-line combination against metastatic disease.

Several European trials having predefined crossover designs and consistency of fluoropyrimidine delivery between arms have further addressed this issue. The GERCOR team in France randomized 220 patients and found that treatment with infusional 5-FU, leucovorin and irinotecan (FOLFIRI) and FOLFOX resulted in comparable response rates and median overall survival times (see Figure 4.19).[68] Similarly, Colucci et al randomized 360 patients to either FOLFOX or FOLFIRI with crossover to the other treatment arm as second-line therapy and found no appreciable difference in response rate, time to progression or overall survival.[95] The consistency of the results suggests equivalence between irinotecan- and oxaliplatin-based regimens when combined with comparable fluorouracil therapies (see Table 4.3).

In addition to combinations of cytotoxic agents, bevacizumab is commonly added to first-line therapy regimens.[88,90] Certain patients should not be exposed to bevacizumab, particularly those at high risk of cardiovascular events. Additionally, bevacizumab can impair wound healing and thus should be avoided in the immediate perioperative period (though an ideal time frame has not been defined, patients should not be exposed to bevacizumab at least 4–6 weeks prior to and after surgery).

Cetuximab and panitumumab were initially tested in patients with prior exposure to other chemotherapies. Randomized trials are ongoing to determine the role of these EGFR inhibitors as part of combination regimens in chemo-naïve patients. At this time, these agents have a role after progression on a prior chemotherapy regimen.

Thus, at present, the optimal sequence of these chemotherapy agents is unclear. The choice of initial therapy could depend on a given patient's baseline comorbidities. For example, irinotecan-based regimens

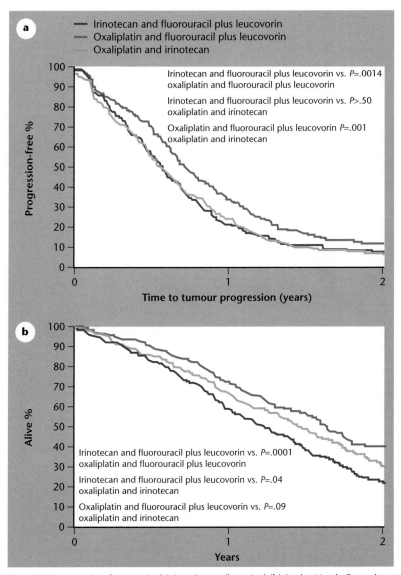

Fig. 4.18 Progression-free survival (**a**) and overall survival (**b**) in the North Central Cancer Treatment Group (NCCTG) 9741. North American trial comparing bolus irinotecan, 5-fluorouracil and leucovorin (IFL) to infusional 5-fluorouracil, leucovorin and oxaliplatin (FOLFOX) to irinotecan and oxaliplatin. Reproduced from Goldberg RM, Sargent DJ, Morton RF, et al: A randomized controlled trial of fluorouracil plus leucovorin, irinotecan, and oxaliplatin combinations in patients with previously untreated metastatic colorectal cancer. J Clin Oncol 2004; 22: 23–30. Reprinted with permission from the American Society of Clinical Oncology.

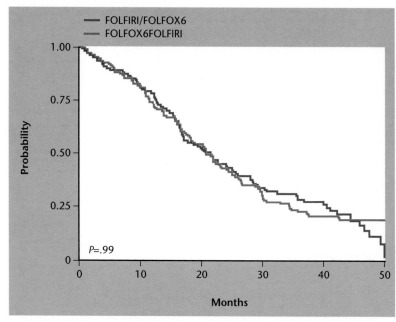

Fig. 4.19 Comparison of irinotecan and oxaliplatin with similar fluoropyrimidine regimens. European study of infusional 5-fluorouracil (5-FU), leucovorin and oxaliplatin (FOLFOX) compared with infusional 5-FU, leucovorin and irinotecan (FOLFIRI) with crossover to opposite treatment as second-line therapy. Reproduced from Tournigand C, Andre T, Achille E, et al: FOLFIRI followed by FOLFOX6 or the reverse sequence in advanced colorectal cancer: a randomized GERCOR study. J Clin Oncol 2004; 22: 229–237. Reprinted with permission from the American Society of Clinical Oncology.

may be more appropriate for a patient who has an underlying neuropathy (avoiding the neurotoxicity of oxaliplatin) while oxaliplatin-based therapy may be more appropriate for patients with underlying bowel dysfunction (avoiding the gastrointestinal toxicity of irinotecan).

STAGE II COLON CANCER

No single randomized clinical trial has demonstrated a survival benefit for adjuvant therapy in patients with stage II colon cancer. In addition, subset analyses of trials that included patients with stage II and III disease have repeatedly failed to demonstrate a statistically significant survival benefit for stage II patients. Combined results from seven studies demonstrated a

Table 4.3 Comparative trials of irinotecan and oxaliplatin as first-line therapy for metastatic colorectal cancer

Trial and interventions	Number of patients	Response rate	Median time to progression (months)	Median overall survival (months)
Goldberg et al[94]				
Irinotecan/bolus 5-FU/LV (IFL) *	264	31%	7.0	15.0
Oxaliplatin/5-FU/LV (FOLFOX)	267	45% (p=0.0001†)	9.3 (p=0.002†)	19.5 (p=0.0001†)
Irinotecan/oxaliplatin	264	35% (p=0.34†)	6.5 (p=0.5†)	17.4 (p=0.04†)
Tournigand et al[68] ‡				
Irinotecan/infusional 5-FU/LV (FOLFIRI)	109	56%	8.5	21.5
Oxaliplatin/infusional 5-FU/LV (FOLFOX6)	111	54% (p=NS)	8.0 (p=0.3)	20.6 (p=0.99)
Colucci et al[95] ‡				
Irinotecan/infusional 5-FU/LV (FOLFIRI)	178	56%	7	14
Oxaliplatin/infusional 5-FU/LV (FOLFOX4)	182	62% (p=NS)	7 (p=0.6)	15 (p=0.3)

5-FU, 5-fluorouracil; LV, leucovorin; NS, not significant
* Control arm
† Compared with control arm (IFL)
‡ In Tournigand et al[68] patients crossed over to the other arm at time of progression of disease or intolerance to first-line therapy. Only the results of trials of first-line therapy are included.

5-year overall survival of 81% in patients who received fluorouracil-based adjuvant therapy and 80% in patients who underwent surgery alone.[96]

Two studies are often cited as demonstrating benefit for adjuvant therapy in stage II disease. A retrospective subset analysis of four consecutive National Surgical Adjuvant Breast and Bowel Project (NSABP) trials demonstrated a similar proportional survival benefit for stage II and stage III patients who received fluorouracil-based therapy.[97] However, the meta-analysis has been faulted by the heterogeneity of the cohorts included, where two trials did not have a surgery-only control arm. The Quick and Simple and Reliable (QUASAR) study also suggested a benefit for patients with stage II disease treated with one of four fluorouracil-based regimens.[98] After median follow-up of 4.6 years, an increase in overall survival was noted for the patients receiving adjuvant therapy (77.3% vs. 80.3%, p=0.02), though 29% of these patients had rectal cancer and 8% did not have stage II disease.

After systematic review of the literature, authors participating in the Cancer Care Ontario Program in Evidence-Based Care recently concluded that "there is no compelling evidence to advise standard use of systemic adjuvant therapy for patients with stage II resected colon cancer".[99] An expert panel convened by the American Society of Clinical Oncology (ASCO) concluded that direct evidence from clinical trials does not support the routine use of adjuvant therapy in patients with stage II colon cancer and that the absolute survival benefit in these patients is unlikely to exceed 5%.[100] In addition, the panel determined that a sample size of 9,680 patients per arm would be required to detect a 2% survival difference between treatment and control arms (90% power with a significance level of 0.05). Finally, the National Comprehensive Cancer Network (NCCN), a consortium of 20 cancer centres that regularly evaluate evidence for treatment of multiple tumour types, does not suggest a universal recommendation of adjuvant chemotherapy for all patients with resected stage II colon cancer.[101]

Although prospective data are lacking, a benefit for adjuvant therapy has been suggested in patients with stage II colon cancer with high-risk features, such as inadequate lymph node sampling, lymphovascular or perineural invasion, T4 tumour stage, clinical colonic perforation or obstruction, and poorly differentiated histology.[20] Though these features may indicate an increased risk of recurrence, they do not necessarily predict for efficacy of chemotherapy. Nonetheless, patients with high-risk stage II colon cancer should be considered for adjuvant therapy.

RADIATION THERAPY

In general, radiation therapy has a more limited role in the treatment of CRC than other solid tumour types. Radiation is often utilized for patients with locally advanced rectal cancer. Radiation may be necessary for palliation of certain specific sites of disease in patients with metastatic CRC (e.g. spinal metastases). Finally, some patients with locally invasive colon cancers may benefit for the addition of radiation to standard chemotherapy.

Anatomically, the rectum is located within the pelvis and extends approximately 12 cm from the transitional mucosa of the dentate line to the sigmoid colon at the peritoneal reflection. The bony constraints of the pelvis limit surgical access to the rectum, leading to a lower likelihood of achieving widely negative margins and a higher risk of local recurrence. To reduce the risk of local recurrence, radiation therapy was incorporated as an adjunct to surgery in resectable rectal cancer.

In Europe, clinical trials evaluated radiation administered prior to surgery in 5 Gy fractions for 5 days. The Swedish Rectal Cancer Trial group randomized 1,168 patients with resectable rectal cancers to receive this "short" course of preoperative radiotherapy (25 Gy in 5 fractions) prior to surgery or surgery alone.[102] The recurrence rate was reduced from 27% to 11% (p<0.001) and the survival was increased from 48% to 58% at 5 years (p=0.004). With the advent of TME surgery, the Dutch Colorectal Cancer Group sought to confirm the role of radiation therapy for rectal cancer.[103] In a preoperative radiotherapy study, 1,861 patients with resectable rectal cancer were randomized to TME surgery alone or five fractions of 5 Gy preoperative radiation followed by TME surgery. The local recurrence at 2 years was 8.2% with surgery alone; however, it was significantly reduced with neoadjuvant radiation (2.8%, p<0.001).

In North America, radiation was more commonly delivered postoperatively as daily 1.8 Gy fractions for 28 treatments. Local control was also improved with the addition of radiation after surgery. The Colorectal Cancer Collaborative Group (CCCG) performed a meta-analysis of 8,507 patients from 22 randomized trials of radiation therapy.[104] At 5 years, preoperative radiation was associated with a significantly lower risk of isolated local recurrence (12.5% vs. 22.2%). For postoperative radiation, the CCCG meta-analysis also demonstrated a significant reduction in the rate of isolated local recurrence (15.3% vs. 22.9%). Although local control was improved with either preoperative or postoperative treatment, neither schedule of radiotherapy was found to provide a significant overall survival advantage compared with surgery alone.

Several randomized, multi-institutional studies published in the late 1980s and early 1990s established combined postoperative chemotherapy and radiation as the standard of care for patients with resected stage II or III rectal cancer.[105–108] The Gastrointestinal Tumor Study Group (GITSG) randomized 227 patients with resected T3–4 and node-positive rectal adenocarcinoma to one of four treatment arms; observation, radiation alone, chemotherapy alone and combined chemoradiation with fluorouracil.[105,106] Combined modality therapy resulted in a statistically significant reduction in local recurrence and increase in overall survival when compared with surgery alone, whereas adjuvant therapy with either chemotherapy or radiation alone did not.[105] A subsequent NCCTG trial also demonstrated a statistically significant improvement in local control and overall survival with combined modality therapy.[107] Due to the improvement in local control and overall survival in these two studies, a National Cancer Institute consensus conference in 1990 recommended the use of adjuvant chemotherapy and radiation for stage II and III rectal cancer.[24] Subsequent studies demonstrated that continuous-infusion fluorouracil was associated with a significantly lower risk of tumour recurrence and an improvement in overall survival.[108]

Investigations into the benefit of neoadjuvant chemoradiation were based on the hope of increasing the possibility of sphincter-preserving surgery with avoidance of a permanent colostomy, and of reducing gastrointestinal toxicity, since less small bowel would be located in the radiation field at the time of treatment. Several phase II trials suggested favourable outcomes with neoadjuvant therapy. Ultimately, the German Rectal Cancer Study Group published a randomized trial of preoperative versus postoperative therapy in 823 patients with T3–4 or node-positive rectal cancer.[1] Patients randomized to preoperative therapy received chemoradiotherapy followed by surgery followed by further adjuvant therapy. Patients randomized to receive surgery as initial treatment received both phases of therapy postoperatively. The German Rectal Cancer Study Group reported that neoadjuvant chemoradiotherapy increased the likelihood of sphincter-sparing surgery and lowered the rates of local recurrence, acute toxicity and long-term toxicity. There were no differences in disease-free or overall survival between the two treatment arms (see Figure 4.20). Although all patients underwent a preoperative endorectal ultrasound, nearly 20% of patients who had up-front surgery were found to have stage I disease on pathological review of the surgical specimen. Thus, it is likely that approximately 20% of patients in the neoadjuvant treatment arm were 'over'-treated. An ongoing Medical Research Council study is evaluating a short course of preoperative radiotherapy against a long course of postoperative chemoradiotherapy for patients with

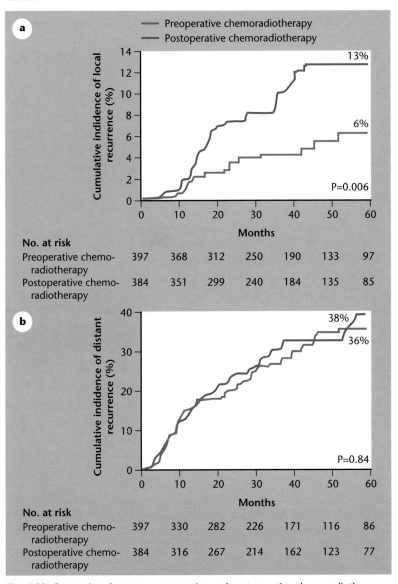

Fig. 4.20 Comparison between preoperative and postoperative chemoradiotherapy in patients with clinical stage II and III rectal cancer. Patients receiving preoperative therapy experienced a lower rate of local recurrences (**a**) and a lower rate of permanent colostomy (**b**) without any differences in disease-free or overall survival. Reproduced with permission from Sauer R, Becker H, Hohenberger W, et al: Preoperative versus postoperative chemoradiotherapy for rectal cancer. N Engl J Med 2004; 351: 1731–1740. © Massachusetts Medical Society.

a mobile, operable tumour that is present within 1 mm of the circumferential resection margin; all surgeries will be TME.

Although no randomized clinical trial has definitively demonstrated the benefit of adjuvant chemotherapy in addition to chemoradiation and surgery in stage II and III rectal cancer, adjuvant chemotherapy is standardly administered to these patients. Few clinical trials have specifically addressed the benefits of adjuvant chemotherapy. EORTC 22921 evaluated the addition of chemotherapy after preoperative radiation therapy that was delivered with or without chemotherapy.[109] With median follow-up of 5.4 years, adjuvant chemotherapy resulted in a non-statistically significant improvement in overall survival (67.2% vs. 63.2%, p=0.12) and progression-free survival (58.2% vs. 52.2%, p=0.13). Further follow-up will be required to evaluate a late divergence seen between the two arms in both endpoints. Data from ongoing studies are required to better define the optimal adjuvant chemotherapy after chemoradiotherapy and surgery in stage II and III rectal cancer.

The role of adjuvant radiation in patients with resected colon cancer is unclear. Patients with positive resection margins or T4 disease (particularly perforation of the visceral peritoneum or invasion of other adjacent organs)[110] are at considerably higher risk for local recurrence than other colon cancer patients. For this reason, adjuvant radiation in addition to chemotherapy has been considered for such select patients. Retrospective data suggest that these patients may benefit from adjuvant radiation.[111] The only available randomized trial, Intergroup 0130, randomly assigned 222 patients with high-risk tumours (adherence to or invasion of adjacent structures or T3 N1–2 tumours of the ascending or descending colon) to fluorouracil chemotherapy with or without adjuvant radiation. Unfortunately, the trial closed due to poor accrual after enrolling only 222 patients (the goal was 700) and, of those patients, 16% were considered ineligible. With these important caveats, there was no significant difference in overall or event-free survival between the two groups at a median follow-up of over 6 years.[112]

LONG-TERM FOLLOW-UP OF PATIENTS

Following surgical resection plus or minus adjuvant therapy, patients with non-metastatic CRC should have regular follow-up with their treating physicians. Despite multiple attempts at addressing the question of optimal follow-up strategies, no single trial has adequately determined which tests and what frequency of tests should be applied for all patients (see Table 4.4).[113–118] Since the majority of recurrences will occur in the

Table 4.4 Randomized trials comparing intensive follow-up to less intensive follow-up after treatment for nonmetastatic colorectal cancer

	Number of patients	Intensive follow-up group	Control group follow-up	Recurrence	Curative attempts *	Survival
Ohlsson et al[113]	107	• Physical exam, rigid proctosigmoidoscopy, CEA, alkaline phosphatase, gamma-glutamyltransferase, haemoglobin, chest X-ray every 3 months x 2 years then every 6 months x 2 years then every year x 1 year • Flexible sigmoidoscopy or colonoscopy of anastomosis at 9, 21, 42 months • Complete colonoscopy at 3, 15, 30, 60 months • CT of pelvis (APR patients only) at 3, 6, 12, 18, 24 months	• Written instructions recommending follow-up every 3 months x 2 years and then yearly faecal occult blood card screenings • Contact physician with symptoms	Int. 32% vs Cont. 33%	Int. 9.4% vs Cont. 5.5%	Int. 75% vs vs Cont. 67% at 5 years (p=0.26)
Makela et al[114]	106	• History, physical exam, complete blood count, faecal occult blood test, CEA, chest X-ray every 3 months x 2 years then every 6 months x 3 years • Colonoscopy at 3 months and then every year • Flexible fibresigmoidoscopy every 3 months (rectal and sigmoid tumours) • Ultrasonography every 6 months • CT of abdomen every year	• History, physical, complete blood count, faecal occult blood test, CEA, chest X-ray every 3 months x 2 years then every 6 months x 3 years • Rigid sigmoidoscopy every patient visit (rectal and sigmoid tumours only) • Barium enema every year	Int. 42% vs Cont. 41%	Int. 9.6% vs Cont. 5.6%	Int. 59% vs Cont. 54% at 5 years (p=0.5)

Table 4.4 Continued Randomized trials comparing intensive follow-up to less intensive follow-up after treatment for nonmetastatic colorectal cancer

	Number of patients	Intensive follow-up group	Control group follow-up	Recurrence	Curative attempts *	Survival
Kjeldsen et al[115]	597	• History, physical exam, digital rectal examination, gynaecological examination, faecal occult blood test, colonoscopy, chest X-ray, haemoglobin, erythrocyte sedimentation rate, liver enzymes at 6, 12, 18, 24, 30, 36, 48, 60, 120, 150, 180 months	• Same as intensive follow-up but at 60, 120, 180 months only	Int. 26% vs Cont. 26%	Int. 22% vs Cont. 7%	Int. 70% vs Cont. 68% at 5 years (p=0.48)
Pietra et al[116]	207	• Physical exam, ultrasound, CEA every 3 months x 2 years then every 6 months x 3 years then every year • Chest X-ray, colonoscopy and CT scan every year	• Physical, ultrasound, CEA every 6 months x 2 years then every year • Chest X-ray, colonoscopy scan every year	Int. 25% vs Cont. 19% (local recurrence) Int. 20% vs Cont. 14% (distant recurrence)	Int. 16% vs Cont. 2% (local recurrence) Int. 3.8% vs Cont. 3.9% (distant recurrence)	Int. 73% vs Cont. 58% at 5 years (p=0.02)
Schoemaker et al[117]	325	• History, physical exam, complete blood count, liver function tests, CEA, faecal occult blood every 3 months x 2 years then every 6 months x 3 years • Chest X-ray, CT liver, colonoscopy every year	• History, physical exam, complete blood count, liver function tests, CEA, faecal occult blood every 3 months x 2 years then every 6 months x 3 years	Int. 34% vs Cont. 40%	Int. 3.6% vs Cont. 3.2%	Int. 74% vs Cont. 65% at 5 years (p=0.2)

Table 4.4 *Continued* **Randomized trials comparing intensive follow-up to less intensive follow-up after treatment for nonmetastatic colorectal cancer**

	Number of patients	Intensive follow-up group	Control group follow-up	Recurrence	Curative attempts *	Survival
Secco et al[118]	337	**High-risk patients** • History, physical exam, CEA every 3 months for 2 years, every 4 months in the third year and every 6 months in years 4 and 5 • Abdominal and pelvic ultrasound performed every 6 months the first 3 year and yearly in years 4 and 5 • Rigid rectosigmoidoscopy and chest X-ray yearly for patients with rectal cancer **Low-risk patients** • History, physical exam, CEA every 6 months for 2 year, then yearly • Abdominal and pelvic ultrasound every 6 months for 2 years, then once a year • Rigid rectosigmoidoscopy for rectal cancer yearly twice, then every 2 years and chest x-ray yearly	• Patients phone surgical team every 6 months and yearly visit with family physician or if symptoms of recurrence appear	Int. 53% vs Cont. 57%	p<0.05 for attempted resections with intensive follow-up	Int. 63% vs Cont. 48% at 5 years (p<0.05)

CEA, carcinoembryonic antigen; CT, computed tomography; APR, abdominoperineal resection; Int, intensive follow-up programme; Cont, control group
* % of all patients in that cohort that underwent curative resection

first 2–3 years after surgery and nearly all recurrences within 5 years, follow-up should be more frequent in the first few years and continue until at least 5 years post-resection. The most common surveillance tools that are recommended and being utilized include physician visits, CEA monitoring, colonoscopic surveillance and additional sigmoidoscopies for rectal cancer patients. Conversely, there is general agreement that liver function tests and complete blood counts are not useful in detecting cancer recurrences. The main controversy has been on the utility and frequency of imaging, including chest X-rays, CT scans or liver ultrasound. Until recently, major oncology organizations have not recommended universal imaging in the absence of symptoms or abnormal CEA testing. However, three meta-analyses of the above-mentioned randomized trials have concluded that more intensive surveillance (which has generally included radiology imaging) provides a modest but statistically significant survival advantage over less intensive surveillance (see Table 4.5).[119–121]

Based on these meta-analyses, ASCO recently updated their guidelines for surveillance of stage II or III colon and rectal cancer patients.[122] An expert panel recommended history and physical examination every 3–6 months for the first 3 years; every 6 months during years 4 and 5, and subsequently at the discretion of the physician; and every 3 months postoperatively for at least 3 years after diagnosis. In addition, for patients who would undergo surgery for metastases, the panel recommended annual CT of the chest and abdomen for 3 years and pelvic CT scan for patients with rectal cancer. The group suggested a colonoscopy 3 years after resection and, if normal, every 5 years thereafter. For patients with rectal cancer who underwent a low anterior resection and did not undergo radiation, more frequency sigmoidoscopies (every 6 months for 5 years) should be considered. It should be noted that an initial colonoscopy is often recommended by other organizations sooner than 3 years since there is a definitive, albeit low, risk of an adenoma or second CRC missed at the time of diagnosis before surgery.

The NCCN has outlined similar recommendations to the ASCO panel, though with more definitive frequency guidelines.[101] NCCN suggests history, physical exam and CEA testing every 3 months for 2 years and then every 6 months for the next 3 years. The group does suggest a colonoscopy at 1 year after surgery, and then either 1 year later if abnormal or every 2–3 years if negative. They suggest consideration of CT scans annually for 3 years, though are less firm than ASCO in recommending such testing. They specifically do not recommend routine PET scan screening. In contrast, the European Society of Medical Oncology

Table 4.5 Meta-analyses of colorectal cancer post-treatment surveillance randomized clinical trials

Meta-analysis	No. of articles analyzed	Pooled no. of patients across trials		Pooled 5-year mortality rate						Effect on 5-year mortality		
		Control	Intervention	Control		Intervention		Absolute risk difference				
				%	No. of patients	%	No. of patients	%	95% CI		95% CI	P
Figueredo et al[119]	6	821	858	37	306 of 821	30	260 of 858	7	3 to 12	Relative risk = 0.80	0.70 to 0.91	0.0008
Renehan et al[120]	5	676	666	37	247 of 666	30	197 of 676	7	2 to 12	Relative risk = 0.81	0.70 to 0.94	0.007
Jeffery et al[121]	5	676	666	37	247 of 666	30	197 of 676	7	2 to 12	Odds ratio = 0.67*	0.53 to 0.84	

*This odds ratio of 0.67 is equivalent to a relative risk of 0.81 for these data

Reproduced with permission from Desch CE, Benson AB 3rd, Somerfield MR, et al: Colorectal cancer surveillance: 2005 update of an American Society of Clinical Oncology practice guideline. J Clin Oncol 2005; 23: 8512–8519

(ESMO) states that radiological examinations are of unproven benefit though they do recommend ultrasonography of the liver every 6 months for 3 years and after 4 and 5 years.[123] ESMO does recommend a colonoscopy at year 1 and then every 3 years thereafter as well as more frequent sigmoidoscopies.

CONCLUSIONS

CRC is a common disease with a significant morbidity and mortality worldwide. It is one of the most understood cancers in terms of factors that alter a subject's risk of developing the disease. These data provide the basis to test preventative strategies, which continues to be a very exciting and active area of research. In addition, therapies against CRC continue to advance (see Figure 4.21). Though screening for CRC remains an essential component to improving survival (both to prevent disease and detect earlier-stage disease), advances in treatment have made appreciable differences over the past several decades. Newer targeted agents are rapidly entering clinical testing and increasing molecular characterizations of tumours should further advance treatment options in the near future.

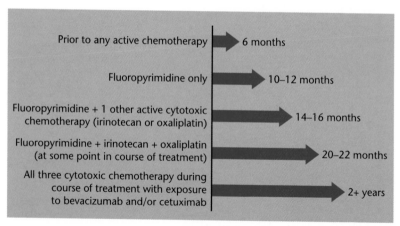

Fig. 4.21 Trends in median survival of patients with advanced colorectal cancer.

REFERENCES

1. Sauer R, Becker H, Hohenberger W, et al: Preoperative versus postoperative chemoradiotherapy for rectal cancer. N Engl J Med 2004; 351: 1731–1740.

2. Nelson H, Petrelli N, Carlin A, et al: Guidelines 2000 for colon and rectal cancer surgery. J Natl Cancer Inst 2001; 93: 583–596.

3. Mehta PP, Griffin J, Ganta S, et al: Laparoscopic-assisted colon resections: long-term results and survival. JSLS 2005; 9: 184–188.

4. The Clinical Outcomes of Surgical Therapy Study Group: A comparison of laparoscopically assisted and open colectomy for colon cancer. N Engl J Med 2004; 350: 2050–2059.

5. Lacy AM, Garcia-Valdecasas JC, Delgado S, et al: Laparoscopy-assisted colectomy versus open colectomy for treatment of non-metastatic colon cancer: a randomised trial. Lancet 2002; 359: 2224–2229.

6. Marr R, Birbeck K, Garvican J, et al: The modern abdominoperineal excision: the next challenge after total mesorectal excision. Ann Surg 2005; 242: 74–82.

7. Khatri VP, Petrelli NJ, Belghiti J: Extending the frontiers of surgical therapy for hepatic colorectal metastases: Is there a limit? J Clin Oncol 2005; 23: 8490–8499.

8. Nordlinger B, Guiguet M, Vaillant JC, et al: Surgical resection of colorectal carcinoma metastases to the liver. A prognostic scoring system to improve case selection, based on 1568 patients. Association Francaise de Chirurgie. Cancer 1996; 77: 1254–1762.

9. Fong Y, Salo J: Surgical therapy of hepatic colorectal metastasis. Semin Oncol 1999; 26: 514–523.

10. Leonard GD, Brenner B, Kemeny NE: Neoadjuvant chemotherapy before liver resection for patients with unresectable liver metastases from colorectal carcinoma. J Clin Oncol 2005; 23: 2038–2048.

11. Giacchetti S, Perpoint B, Zidani R, et al: Phase III multicenter randomized trial of oxaliplatin added to chronomodulated fluorouracil-leucovorin as first-line treatment of metastatic colorectal cancer. J Clin Oncol 2000; 18: 136–147.

12. Folprecht G, Grothey A, Alberts S, et al: Neoadjuvant treatment of unresectable colorectal liver metastases: correlation between tumour response and resection rates. Ann Oncol 2005; 16: 1311–1319.

13. Zhang ZG, Harstrick A, Rustum YM: Modulation of fluoropyrimidines: role of dose and schedule of leucovorin administration. Semin Oncol 1992; 19: 10–15.

14. Scheithauer W, Rosen H, Kornek GV, et al: Randomised comparison of combination chemotherapy plus supportive care with supportive care alone in patients with metastatic colorectal cancer. BMJ 1993; 306: 752–755.

15. Smyth JF, Hardcastle JD, Denton G, et al: Two phase III trials of tauromustine (TCNU) in advanced colorectal cancer. Ann Oncol 1995; 6: 948–949.

16. Allen-Mersh TG, Earlam S, Fordy C, et al: Quality of life and survival with continuous hepatic-artery floxuridine infusion for colorectal liver metastases. Lancet 1994; 344: 1255–1260.

17. Thirion P, Michiels S, Pignon JP, et al: Modulation of fluorouracil by leucovorin in patients with advanced colorectal cancer: an updated meta-analysis. J Clin Oncol 2004; 22: 3766–3775.

18. Laurie JA, Moertel CG, Fleming TR, et al: Surgical adjuvant therapy of large-bowel carcinoma: an evaluation of levamisole and the combination of levamisole and fluorouracil. The North Central Cancer Treatment Group and the Mayo Clinic. J Clin Oncol 1989; 7: 1447–1456.

19. Moertel CG, Fleming TR, Macdonald JS, et al: Levamisole and fluorouracil for adjuvant therapy of resected colon carcinoma. N Engl J Med 1990; 322: 352–358.

20. Moertel CG, Fleming TR, Macdonald JS, et al: Fluorouracil plus levamisole as effective adjuvant therapy after resection of stage III colon carcinoma: a final report. Ann Intern Med 1995; 122: 321–326.

21. Haller DG, Catalano PJ, Macdonald JS, et al: Phase III study of fluorouracil, leucovorin, and levamisole in high-risk stage II and III colon cancer: final report of Intergroup 0089. J Clin Oncol 2005; 23: 8671–8678.

22. QUASAR Collaborative Group: Comparison of flourouracil with additional levamisole, higher-dose folinic acid, or both, as adjuvant chemotherapy for colorectal cancer: a randomised trial. Lancet 2000; 355: 1588–1596.

23. International Multicentre Pooled Analysis of Colon Cancer Trials (IMPACT) investigators: Efficacy of adjuvant fluorouracil and folinic acid in colon cancer. Lancet 1995; 345: 939–944.

24. NIH consensus conference: Adjuvant therapy for patients with colon and rectal cancer. JAMA 1990; 264: 1444–1450.

25. Lokich JJ, Ahlgren JD, Gullo JJ, et al: A prospective randomized comparison of continuous infusion fluorouracil with a conventional bolus schedule in metastatic colorectal carcinoma: a Mid-Atlantic Oncology Program Study. J Clin Oncol 1989; 7: 425–432.

26. de Gramont A, Bosset JF, Milan C, et al: Randomized trial comparing monthly low-dose leucovorin and fluorouracil bolus with bimonthly high-dose leucovorin and fluorouracil bolus plus continuous infusion for advanced colorectal cancer: a French intergroup study. J Clin Oncol 1997; 15: 808–815.

27. Weh HJ, Wilke HJ, Dierlamm J, et al: Weekly therapy with folinic acid (FA) and high-dose 5-fluorouracil (5-FU) 24-hour infusion in pretreated patients with metastatic colorectal carcinoma. A multicenter study by the Association of Medical Oncology of the German Cancer Society (AIO). Ann Oncol 1994; 5: 233–237.

28. Lokich JJ, Moore CL, Anderson NR: Comparison of costs for infusion versus bolus chemotherapy administration: analysis of five standard chemotherapy regimens in three common tumors—Part one. Model projections for cost based on charges. Cancer 1996; 78: 294–299.

29. Kohne CH, Wils J, Lorenz M, et al: Randomized phase III study of high-dose fluorouracil given as a weekly 24-hour infusion with or without leucovorin versus bolus fluorouracil plus leucovorin in advanced colorectal cancer: European organization of Research and Treatment of Cancer Gastrointestinal Group Study 40952. J Clin Oncol 2003; 21: 3721–3718.

30. Efficacy of intravenous continuous infusion of fluorouracil compared with bolus administration in advanced colorectal cancer. Meta-analysis Group In Cancer. J Clin Oncol 1998; 16: 301–308.

31. Hahn RG, Moertel CG, Schutt AJ, et al: A double-blind comparison of intensive course 5-flourouracil by oral vs. intravenous route in the treatment of colorectal carcinoma. Cancer 1975; 35: 1031–1035.

32. Pentheroudakis G, Twelves C: The rational development of capecitabine from the laboratory to the clinic. Anticancer Res 2002; 22: 3589–3596.

33. Meropol NJ: Oral fluoropyrimidines in the treatment of colorectal cancer. Eur J Cancer 1998; 34: 1509–1513.

34. Sulkes A, Benner SE, Canetta RM: Uracil-ftorafur: an oral fluoropyrimidine active in colorectal cancer. J Clin Oncol 1998; 16: 3461–3475.

35. Sakata Y, Ohtsu A, Horikoshi N, et al: Late phase II study of novel oral fluo-ropyrimidine anticancer drug S-1 (1 M tegafur-0.4 M gimestat-1 M otastat potassium) in advanced gastric cancer patients. Eur J Cancer 1998; 34: 1715–1720.

36. Van Cutsem E, Twelves C, Cassidy J, et al: Oral capecitabine compared with intravenous fluorouracil plus leucovorin in patients with metastatic colorectal cancer: results of a large phase III study. J Clin Oncol 2001; 19: 4097–4106.

37. Hoff PM, Ansari R, Batist G, et al: Comparison of oral capecitabine versus intravenous fluorouracil plus leucovorin as first-line treatment in 605 patients with metastatic colorectal cancer: results of a randomized phase III study. J Clin Oncol 2001; 19: 2282–2292.

38. Mayer RJ: Oral versus intravenous fluoropyrimidines for advanced colorec-tal cancer: by either route, it's all the same. J Clin Oncol 2001; 19: 4093–4096.

39. Twelves C, Wong A, Nowacki MP, et al: Capecitabine as adjuvant treatment for stage III colon cancer. N Engl J Med 2005; 352: 2696–2704.

40. Carmichael J, Popiela T, Radstone D, et al: Randomized comparative study of tegafur/uracil and oral leucovorin versus parenteral fluorouracil and leu-covorin in patients with previously untreated metastatic colorectal cancer. J Clin Oncol 2002; 20: 3617–3627.

41. Douillard JY, Hoff PM, Skillings JR, et al: Multicenter phase III study of uracil/tegafur and oral leucovorin versus fluorouracil and leucovorin in patients with previously untreated metastatic colorectal cancer. J Clin Oncol 2002; 20: 3605–3616.

42. Wolmark N, Wieand HS, Kuebler JP, Colangelo L, Smith RE: A phase III trial comparing FULV to FULV + oxaliplatin in stage II or III carcinoma of the colon: Results of NSABP protocol C-07. J Clin Oncol 2005; 23 Suppl: 3500 abstract.

43. Iyer L, Ratain MJ: Clinical pharmacology of camptothecins. Cancer Chemother Pharmacol 1998; 42 Suppl: S31–S43.

44. Klein CE, Gupta E, Reid JM, et al: Population pharmacokinetic model for irinotecan and two of its metabolites, SN-38 and SN-38 glucuronide. Clin Pharmacol Ther 2002; 72: 638–647.

45. Mathijssen RH, van Alphen RJ, Verweij J, et al: Clinical pharmacokinetics and metabolism of irinotecan (CPT-11). Clin Cancer Res 2001; 7: 2182–2194.

46. Iyer L, Das S, Janisch L, et al: UGT1A1*28 polymorphism as a determinant of irinotecan disposition and toxicity. Pharmacogenomics J 2002; 2: 43–47.

47. Ando Y, Saka H, Asai G, et al: UGT1A1 genotypes and glucuronidation of SN-38, the active metabolite of irinotecan. Ann Oncol 1998; 9: 845–847.

48. Innocenti F, Undevia SD, Iyer L, et al: Genetic variants in the UDP-glu-curonosyltransferase 1A1 gene predict the risk of severe neutropenia of irinotecan. J Clin Oncol 2004; 22: 1382–1388.

49. Rougier P, Van Cutsem E, Bajetta E, et al: Randomised trial of irinotecan versus fluorouracil by continuous infusion after fluorouracil failure in patients with metastatic colorectal cancer. Lancet 1998; 352: 1407–1412.

50. Cunningham D, Pyrhonen S, James RD, et al: Randomised trial of irinote-can plus supportive care versus supportive care alone after fluorouracil fail-ure for patients with metastatic colorectal cancer. Lancet 1998; 352: 1413–1418.

51. Douillard JY, Cunningham D, Roth AD, et al: Irinotecan combined with fluorouracil compared with fluorouracil alone as first-line treatment for metastatic colorectal cancer: a multicentre randomised trial. Lancet 2000; 355: 1041–1047.

52. Saltz LB, Cox JV, Blanke C, et al: Irinotecan plus fluorouracil and leucovorin for metastatic colorectal cancer. Irinotecan Study Group. N Engl J Med 2000; 343: 905–914.

53. Saltz LB, Niedzwiecki D, Hollis D, et al: Irinotecan plus fluorouracil/leucovorin (IFL) versus fluorouracil/leucovorin alone (FL) in stage III colon cancer (intergroup trial CALGB C89803). J Clin Oncol 2004 ASCO Annual Meeting Proceedings 22:3500.

54. Van Cutsem E, Labianca R, Hossfeld D, Bodoky G, et al: Randomized phase III trial comparing infused irinotecan / 5-fluorouracil (5-FU) / folinic acid (IF) versus 5-FU / FA (F) in stage III colon cancer patients (PETACC 3). J Clin Oncol 2005; 23 Suppl: 8 abstract.

55. Ychou MRJ, Douillard J, Bugat R, et al: A phase III randomized trial of LV5FU2+CPT-11 vs. LV5FU2 alone in adjuvant high risk colon cancer (FNCLCC Accord02/FFCD9802). J Clin Oncol 2005; 23 Suppl: 3502 abstract.

56. Raymond E, Faivre S, Woynarowski JM, et al: Oxaliplatin: mechanism of action and antineoplastic activity. Semin Oncol 1998; 25: 4–12.

57. Rixe O, Ortuzar W, Alvarez M, et al: Oxaliplatin, tetraplatin, cisplatin, and carboplatin: spectrum of activity in drug-resistant cell lines and in the cell lines of the National Cancer Institute's Anticancer Drug Screen panel. Biochem Pharmacol 1996; 52: 1855–1865.

58. Raymond E, Buquet-Fagot C, Djelloul S, et al: Antitumor activity of oxaliplatin in combination with 5-fluorouracil and the thymidylate synthase inhibitor AG337 in human colon, breast and ovarian cancers. Anticancer Drugs 1997; 8: 876–885.

59. Rothenberg ML, Oza AM, Bigelow RH, et al: Superiority of oxaliplatin and fluorouracil-leucovorin compared with either therapy alone in patients with progressive colorectal cancer after irinotecan and fluorouracil-leucovorin: interim results of a phase III trial. J Clin Oncol 2003; 21: 2059–2069.

60. Raymond E, Faivre S, Chaney S, et al: Cellular and molecular pharmacology of oxaliplatin. Mol Cancer Ther 2002; 1: 227–235.

61. Grothey A: Oxaliplatin-safety profile: neurotoxicity. Semin Oncol 2003; 30: 5–13.

62. de Gramont A, Figer A, Seymour M, et al: Leucovorin and fluorouracil with or without oxaliplatin as first-line treatment in advanced colorectal cancer. J Clin Oncol 2000; 18: 2938–2947.

63. Becouarn Y, Ychou M, Ducreux M, et al: Phase II trial of oxaliplatin as first-line chemotherapy in metastatic colorectal cancer patients. Digestive Group of French Federation of Cancer Centers. J Clin Oncol 1998; 16: 2739–2744.

64. Diaz-Rubio E, Sastre J, Zaniboni A, et al: Oxaliplatin as single agent in previously untreated colorectal carcinoma patients: a phase II multicentric study. Ann Oncol 1998; 9: 105–108.

65. Levi F, Perpoint B, Garufi C, et al: Oxaliplatin activity against metastatic colorectal cancer. A phase II study of 5-day continuous venous infusion at circadian rhythm modulated rate. Eur J Cancer 1993; 29A: 1280–1284.

66. Machover D, Diaz-Rubio E, de Gramont A, et al: Two consecutive phase II studies of oxaliplatin (L-OHP) for treatment of patients with advanced colorectal carcinoma who were resistant to previous treatment with fluoropyrimidines. Ann Oncol 1996; 7: 95–98.

67. Grothey A, Deschler B, Kroening H, et al: Phase III study of bolus 5-fluo-rouracil (5-FU)/ folinic acid (FA) (Mayo) vs weekly high-dose 24h 5-FU infu-sion/ FA + oxaliplatin (OXA) (FUFOX) in advanced colorectal cancer (ACRC). Proc Am Soc Clin Oncol 2002; 21: 129a.

68. Tournigand C, Andre T, Achille E, et al: FOLFIRI followed by FOLFOX6 or the reverse sequence in advanced colorectal cancer: a randomized GERCOR study. J Clin Oncol 2004; 22: 229–237.

69. Andre T, Boni C, Mounedji-Boudiaf L, et al: Oxaliplatin, fluorouracil, and leucovorin as adjuvant treatment for colon cancer. N Engl J Med 2004; 350: 2343–2351.

70. De Gramont A BC, Navarro M, Tabernero J, et al: Oxaliplatin/ 5FU/ LV in the adjuvant treatment of stage II and III colon cancer: efficacy results with a median follow-up of 4 years. J Clin Oncol 2005; 23 Suppl: 3501 abstract.

71. Baselga J, Albanell J: Epithelial growth factor receptor interacting agents. Hematol Oncol Clin North Am 2002; 16: 1041–1063.

72. Spaulding DC, Spaulding BO: Epidermal growth factor receptor expression and measurement in solid tumors. Semin Oncol 2002; 29: 45–54.

73. Messa C, Russo F, Caruso MG, et al: EGF, TGF-alpha, and EGF-R in human colorectal adenocarcinoma. Acta Oncol 1998; 37: 285–289.

74. Porebska I, Harlozinska A, Bojarowski T: Expression of the tyrosine kinase activity growth factor receptors (EGFR, ERB B2, ERB B3) in colorectal adeno-carcinomas and adenomas. Tumour Biol 2000; 21: 105–115.

75. Mayer A, Takimoto M, Fritz E, et al: The prognostic significance of prolifer-ating cell nuclear antigen, epidermal growth factor receptor, and mdr gene expression in colorectal cancer. Cancer 1993; 71: 2454–2460.

76. Venook AP: Epidermal growth factor receptor-targeted treatment for advanced colorectal carcinoma. Cancer 2005; 103: 2435–2446.

77. Rothenberg ML, LaFleur B, Levy DE, et al: Randomized phase II trial of the clinical and biological effects of two dose levels of gefitinib in patients with recurrent colorectal adenocarcinoma. J Clin Oncol 2005; 23: 9265–9274.

78. Blanke CD: Gefitinib in colorectal cancer: if wishes were horses. J Clin Oncol 2005; 23: 5446–5449.

79. Prewett MC, Hooper AT, Bassi R, et al: Enhanced antitumor activity of anti-epidermal growth factor receptor monoclonal antibody IMC-C225 in com-bination with irinotecan (CPT-11) against human colorectal tumor xenografts. Clin Cancer Res 2002; 8: 994–1003.

80. Saltz L, Rubin M, Hochster H, et al: Cetuximab (IMC-C225) plus irinotecan (CPT-11) is active in CPT-11-refractory colorectal cancer (CRC) that express-es epidermal growth factor receptor (EGFR). Proc Am Soc Clin Oncol 2001; 20: 3a.

81. Saltz LB, Meropol NJ, Loehrer PJ Sr, et al: Phase II trial of cetuximab in patients with refractory colorectal cancer that expresses the epidermal growth factor receptor. J Clin Oncol 2004; 22: 1201–1208.

82. Cunningham D, Humblet Y, Siena S, et al: Cetuximab monotherapy and cetuximab plus irinotecan in irinotecan-refractory metastatic colorectal can-cer. N Engl J Med 2004; 351: 337–345.

83. Segaert S, Van Cutsem E: Clinical signs, pathophysiology and management of skin toxicity during therapy with epidermal growth factor receptor inhibitors. Ann Oncol 2005; 16: 1425–1433.

84. Malik I, Hecht JR, Patnaik A, et al: Safety and efficacy of panitumumab monotherapy in patients with metastatic colorectal cancer. Proc Am Soc Clin Oncol 2005; 23: Abstract 3520.

85. Abgenix Inc: Panitumumab significantly improves progression-free survival in phase 3 randomized metastatic colorectal cancer study, 2005.

86. Folkman J: Tumor angiogenesis: therapeutic implications. N Engl J Med 1971; 285: 1182–1186.

87. Ferrara N, Gerber HP, LeCouter J: The biology of VEGF and its receptors. Nat Med 2003; 9: 669–676.

88. Kabbinavar F, Hurwitz HI, Fehrenbacher L, et al: Phase II, randomized trial comparing bevacizumab plus fluorouracil (FU)/leucovorin (LV) with FU/LV alone in patients with metastatic colorectal cancer. J Clin Oncol 2003; 21: 60–65.

89. Kabbinavar FF, Schulz J, McCleod M, et al: Addition of bevacizumab to bolus fluorouracil and leucovorin in first-line metastatic colorectal cancer: results of a randomized phase II trial. J Clin Oncol 2005; 23: 3697–3705.

90. Hurwitz H, Fehrenbacher L, Novotny W, et al: Bevacizumab plus irinotecan, fluorouracil, and leucovorin for metastatic colorectal cancer. N Engl J Med 2004; 350: 2335–2342.

91. Giantonio BJ, Catalano PJ, Meropol NJ, et al: High-dose bevacizumab improves survival when combined with FOLFOX4 in previously treated advanced colorectal cancer: Results from the Eastern Cooperative Oncology Group (ECOG) study E3200. Proc Am Soc Clin Oncol 2005; 6: abstract 2.

92. Hochster HS, Hart LL, Ramanathan RK, et al: Safety and efficacy of oxaliplatin/fluoropyrimidine regimens with or without bevacizumab as first-line treatment of metastatic colorectal cancer (mCRC): Final analysis of the TREE-Study. J Clin Oncol, 2006 ASCO Annual Meeting Proceedings Part I; 24: 3510.

93. Grothey A, Sargent D, Goldberg RM, et al: Survival of patients with advanced colorectal cancer improves with the availability of fluorouracil-leucovorin, irinotecan, and oxaliplatin in the course of treatment. J Clin Oncol 2004; 22: 1209–1214.

94. Goldberg RM, Sargent DJ, Morton RF, et al: A randomized controlled trial of fluorouracil plus leucovorin, irinotecan, and oxaliplatin combinations in patients with previously untreated metastatic colorectal cancer. J Clin Oncol 2004; 22: 23–30.

95. Colucci G, Gebbia V, Paoletti G, et al: Phase III randomized trial of FOLFIRI versus FOLFOX4 in the treatment of advanced colorectal cancer: a multicenter study of the Gruppo Oncologico Dell'Italia Meridionale. J Clin Oncol 2005; 23: 4866–4875.

96. Gill S, Loprinzi CL, Sargent DJ, et al: Pooled analysis of fluorouracil-based adjuvant therapy for stage II and III colon cancer: who benefits and by how much? J Clin Oncol 2004; 22: 1797–1806.

97. Mamounas E, Wieand S, Wolmark N, et al: Comparative efficacy of adjuvant chemotherapy in patients with Dukes' B versus Dukes' C colon cancer: results from four National Surgical Adjuvant Breast and Bowel Project adjuvant studies (C-01, C-02, C-03, and C-04). J Clin Oncol 1999; 17: 1349–1355.

98. Gray RG, Hills R, McConkey C, et al: QUASAR: A randomized study of adjuvant chemotherapy (CT) vs observation including 3238 colorectal cancer patients. Proc Am Soc Clin Oncol 2004, Abstract 3501.

99. Figueredo A, Charette ML, Maroun J, et al: Adjuvant therapy for stage II colon cancer: a systematic review from the Cancer Care Ontario Program in evidence-based care's gastrointestinal cancer disease site group. J Clin Oncol 2004; 22: 3395–3407.

100. Benson AB, Schrag D, Somerfield MR, et al: American Society of Clinical Oncology recommendations on adjuvant chemotherapy for stage II colon cancer. J Clin Oncol 2004; 22: 3408–3419.

101. Engstrom P: Update: NCCN colon cancer clinical practice guidelines. J Natl Compr Canc Netw 2005; 3 Suppl 1: S25–S28.

102. Swedish Rectal Cancer Trial: Improved survival with preoperative radiotherapy in resectable rectal cancer. N Engl J Med 1997; 336: 980–987.

103. Kapiteijn E, Marijnen CA, Nagtegaal ID, et al: Preoperative radiotherapy combined with total mesorectal excision for resectable rectal cancer. N Engl J Med 2001; 345: 638–646.

104. Colorectal Cancer Collaborative Group: Adjuvant radiotherapy for rectal cancer: a systematic overview of 8,507 patients from 22 randomised trials. Lancet 2001; 358: 1291–1304.

105. Gastrointestinal Tumor Study Group: Prolongation of the disease-free interval in surgically treated rectal carcinoma. N Engl J Med 1985; 312: 1465–1472.

106. Douglass HO, Jr, Moertel CG, Mayer RJ, et al: Survival after postoperative combination treatment of rectal cancer. N Engl J Med 1986; 315: 1294–1295.

107. Krook JE, Moertel CG, Gunderson LL, et al: Effective surgical adjuvant therapy for high-risk rectal carcinoma. N Engl J Med 1991; 324: 709–715.

108. O'Connell MJ, Martenson JA, Wieand HS, et al: Improving adjuvant therapy for rectal cancer by combining protracted-infusion fluorouracil with radiation therapy after curative surgery. N Engl J Med 1994; 331: 502–507.

109. Bosset JF, Calais G, Mineur L, et al: Enhanced tumorocidal effect of chemotherapy with preoperative radiotherapy for rectal cancer: preliminary results—EORTC 22921. J Clin Oncol 2005; 23: 5620–5627.

110. Willett C, Tepper JE, Cohen A, et al: Obstructive and perforative colonic carcinoma: Patterns of failure. J Clin Oncol 1985; 3: 379–384.

111. Willett CG, Fung CY, Kaufman DS, et al: Postoperative radiation therapy for high-risk colon carcinoma. J Clin Oncol 1993; 11: 1112–1117.

112. Martenson JA, Jr, Willett CG, Sargent DJ, et al: Phase III study of adjuvant chemotherapy and radiation therapy compared with chemotherapy alone in the surgical adjuvant treatment of colon cancer: results of intergroup protocol 0130. J Clin Oncol 2004; 22: 3277–3283.

113. Ohlsson B, Breland U, Ekberg H, et al: Follow-up after curative surgery for colorectal carcinoma. Randomized comparison with no follow-up. Dis Colon Rectum 1995; 38: 619–626.

114. Makela JT, Laitinen SO, Kairaluoma MI: Five-year follow-up after radical surgery for colorectal cancer. Results of a prospective randomized trial. Arch Surg 1995; 130: 1062–1067.

115. Kjeldsen BJ, Kronborg O, Fenger C, et al: A prospective randomized study of follow-up after radical surgery for colorectal cancer. Br J Surg 1997; 84: 666–669.

116. Pietra N, Sarli L, Costi R, et al: Role of follow-up in management of local recurrences of colorectal cancer: a prospective, randomized study. Dis Colon Rectum 1998; 41: 1127–1133.

117. Schoemaker D, Black R, Giles L, et al: Yearly colonoscopy, liver CT, and chest radiography do not influence 5-year survival of colorectal cancer patients. Gastroenterology 1998; 114: 7–14.

118. Secco GB, Fardelli R, Gianquinto D, et al: Efficacy and cost of risk-adapted follow-up in patients after colorectal cancer surgery: a prospective, randomized and controlled trial. Eur J Surg Oncol 2002; 28: 418–423.

119. Figueredo A, Rumble RB, Maroun J, et al: Follow-up of patients with curatively resected colorectal cancer: A practice guideline. BMC Cancer 2003; 3: 26.

120. Renehan AG, Egger M, Saunders MP, et al: Impact on survival of intensive follow up after curative resection for colorectal cancer: systematic review and meta-analysis of randomised trials. BMJ 2002; 324: 813.

121. Jeffery GM, Hickey BE, Hider P: Follow-up strategies for patients treated for non-metastatic colorectal cancer. Cochrane Database Syst Rev 2002: CD002200.

122. Desch CE, Benson AB, 3rd, Somerfield MR, et al: Colorectal cancer surveillance: 2005 update of an American Society of Clinical Oncology practice guideline. J Clin Oncol 2005; 23: 8512–8519.

123. Van Cutsem EJ, Kataja VV: ESMO minimum clinical recommendations for diagnosis, adjuvant treatment and follow-up of colon cancer. Ann Oncol 2005; 16 Suppl 1: i16–i17.

Systemic and mucocutaneous reactions to chemotherapy

5

Joseph P. Eder and Arthur T. Skarin

Cancer chemotherapy is a major component of cancer therapy, along with surgery and radiation. Cancer chemotherapy agents differ from most drugs in that it is intentionally cytotoxic to human cells. This aspect of cancer chemotherapeutic agents produces a narrow therapeutic index (desired vs. undesired effects) for most, but not all, agents in this class. The target of cancer chemotherapeutic agents is the proliferating cancer cell. While many normal tissues are non-proliferating, some are proliferating and toxicity of this class tends to preferentially overlap proliferating tissues – haematopoietic, gastrointestinal mucosa and skin. In addition, each agent often has specific organ toxicity related to its chemical class or unique mechanism of action.

The major groups of cancer chemotherapeutic agents are the direct-acting alkylating agents, the indirect-acting anthracyclines and topoisomerase inhibitors, the antimetabolites, the tubulin-binding agents, hormones, receptor-targeted agents and a class of miscellaneous agents. Despite the disparate nature of this broad class of agents, some generalizations about the effects of chemotherapy are still possible. For more information readers are referred to detailed reports.[1,2]

ACUTE HYPERSENSITIVITY REACTIONS

Acute hypersensitivity can occur with any drug. However, several cancer chemotherapeutic agents are derived from hydrophobic plant chemicals and must be solubilized with agents with a marked propensity for causing acute hypersensitivity reactions, especially histamine-mediated anaphylactic reactions, such as the Cremophor used with paclitaxel. Docetaxel has a lower incidence of this complication.

The incidence of severe hypersensitivity reactions with paclitaxel may be up to 25% without ancillary measures. With antihistamine H1 and H2 blockade and corticosteroids, the incidence falls to 2–3%. Hypersensitivity reactions occur in up to 40% of patients receiving single agent 1-asparaginase but only 20% when administered in combination therapy with glucocorticoids and 6-mercaptopurine, perhaps as a result of immunosuppression. The hypersensitivity usually occurs after several doses and in successive cycles. The reaction may be only urticaria (see Figure 5.1) but may be severe with laryngospasm or, rarely, serum sickness. Fatal reactions occur <1% of the time. Changing the source of enzyme is the appropriate initial step. Two other proteins in

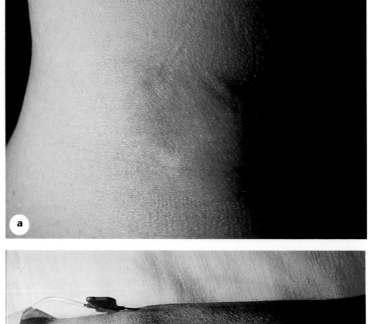

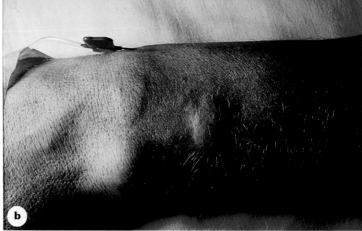

Fig. 5.1 Acute hypersensitivity reactions. Urticaria, with giant localized hives, occurred (**a**) in a 40-year-old man within a few minutes of receiving intravenous 5-fluorouracil and (**b**) in the lower arm of a 50-year-old man after receiving adriamycin. The urticaria was self-limiting in both patients.

clinical use, rituximab and traztuzumab, have a similar incidence of hypersensitivity reactions.

Certain drugs such as etoposide are associated with a greater incidence of reactions but most are not true hypersensitivity reactions. The Tween diluant in the clinical etoposide formulation produces hypotension, rash and back pain. The platinum compounds carboplatin and cisplatin are associated with hypersensitivity reactions, particularly on subsequent cycles – most of these reactions are severe (75%).[3] Hypersensitivity to platinum and related compounds is actually quite frequent, up to 14% in industrial workers, so such reactions in patients receiving these agents parenterally should not be surprising and is often unappreciated in combination chemotherapy regimens, such as with taxanes, and may be equally suppressed by the prophylactic regimens employed.[4] Liposomal encapsulated anthracyclines are associated with an increased incidence of hypersensitivity compared with the parent drugs. Like the reaction to Cremophor EL and radiocontrast agents, the reaction is a "complement activation pseudoallergy".[5] Up to 45% of cancer patients show activation of the classical, alternative or both complement pathways, although the incidence of clinical reactions is about 20%.

Monoclonal antibodies such as trastuzumab, rituximab, bevacizumab, and cetuximab have had enormous impact on cancer therapeutics. Monoclonal antibodies may be chimeric (a murine Fab binding site but human amino acid sequences elsewhere) or fully human. Allergic or hypersensitivity reactions are more frequent with chimeric proteins such as cetuximab (1–5% clinically significant) and are treated with antihistamines and steroids plus slowing of the infusion. L-Asparaginase is a bacterial protein that frequently results in hypersensitivity reactions. These reactions are more frequent with interrupted schedules and with subsequent re-challenge. Changing the source from *Escherichia coli* to *Erwinia* is one accepted strategem if immunosuppression does not work.

ALOPECIA

Many antineoplastic drugs can produce marked hair loss (see Figure 5.2). This includes not only scalp hair but also facial, axillary, pubic and all body hair. The germinating hair follicle has an approximately 24-hour doubling time. Cancer chemotherapy agents preferentially affect actively growing (anagen) hairs. The interruption of mitosis produces a structurally weakened hair prone to fracture easily from minimal trauma such as brushing. Since 80–90% of scalp hairs are in anagen phase, the degree

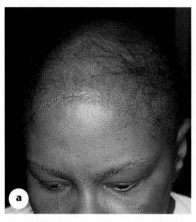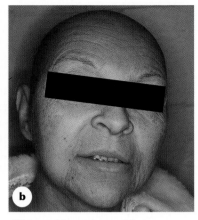

Fig. 5.2 Alopecia. (**a**) Near-total alopecia in a 38-year-old woman receiving cyclophosphamide and adriamycin. Note the loss of eyebrow and eyelid hair. (**b**) Total alopecia developed in this 64-year-old woman due to chemotherapy and cranial irradiation for brain metastases. The duration of alopecia after both treatment modalities may be many months or even permanent in some patients. In this woman, the scalp oedema and erythema are related to an allergic cutaneous reaction from diphenyl hydantoin.

of hair loss can be substantial. Hair loss, while often emotionally difficult for patients, is reversible, although hair may regrow more curly and of a slightly different colour.

STOMATITIS/MUCOSITIS

The oral complications of cancer chemotherapy are many and frequently severe. The disruption of the protective mucosal barrier serves as a portal of entry for pathogens which, especially when combined with chemotherapy-induced neutropenia, predisposes to local infection and systemic sepsis. Once established, these infections may be difficult to eradicate in immunocompromised patients. The most common infectious organisms are *Candida albicans*, herpes simplex virus, β-haemolytic streptococci, staphylococci, opportunistic Gram-negative bacteria and mouth anaerobes.

Several agents of the antimetabolite class of cancer chemotherapeutic agents, especially those that target pyrimidine biosynthesis such as methotrexate, 5-fluorouracil (5-FU) and cytosine arabinoside, and the anthracyline agents, such as doxorubicin and daunorubicin, are particularly toxic to the mucosal epithelium (see Figure 5.3). These agents

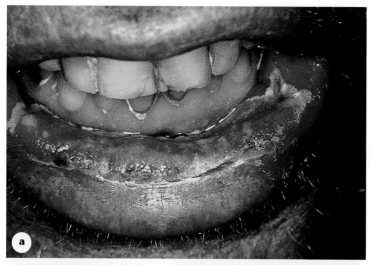

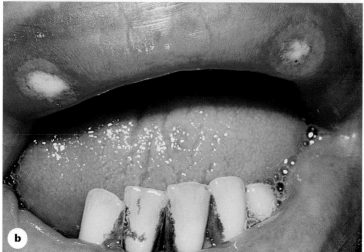

Fig. 5.3 Stomatitis and mucositis. (**a**) Marked stomatitis in a patient receiving methotrexate. (**b**) Aphthous stomatitis related to severe granulocytopenia after chemotherapy. The ulcers may be due to herpes simplex or other infection.

have a marked capacity to produce more severe injury in irradiated tissues, even if the radiation is temporally remote. These agents produce marked ulceration and erosion of the mucosa. These lesions occur initially on those mucosal surfaces that abrade the teeth and gums, such as the sides of the tongue, the vermillion border of the lower lip and the

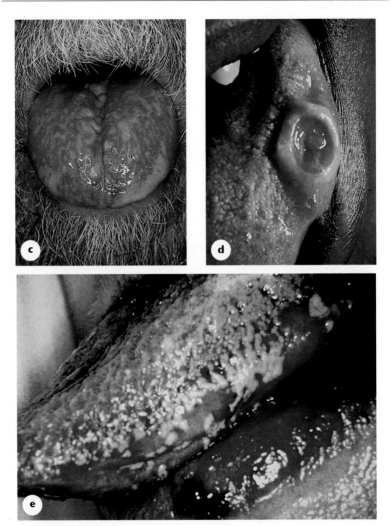

Fig. 5.3 Continued (c) Mucositis in a patient receiving combination chemotherapy for head and neck cancer. **(d)** Marked ulcer of the tongue in a 32-year-old man receiving induction chemotherapy for acute leukaemia. **(e)** Mucositis of the tongue due to monilia infection (thrush) in a patient receiving corticosteroids for brain metastases.

buccal mucosa. More advanced mucosal injury may occur on the hard and soft palate and the posterior oropharynx. These ulcerations cannot often be distinguished from those caused by infectious organisms. Appropriate tests must be performed to exclude viral, fungal and bacterial causes or superinfection.

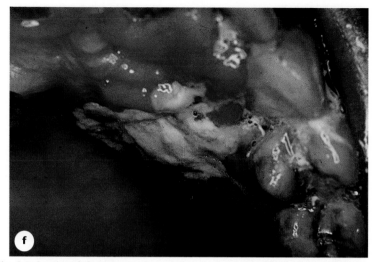

Fig. 5.3 *Continued* (f) Marked oral mucositis due to mixed infection in a patient receiving chemotherapy for acute leukaemia.

In addition to the risk of infection, the resultant pain makes patients unable to maintain adequate nutrition and hydration. This may compromise the capacity to complete a course of chemotherapy and require prolonged administration of parenteral fluids and even parenteral nutrition.

DERMATITIS, SKIN RASHES AND HYPERPIGMENTATION

Superficial manifestations of cancer chemotherapy agents are noted frequently by patients, although they are considered significant much less often by clinicians. The cosmetic changes may be disturbing to patients without requiring discontinuation of therapy.

Of the direct-acting alkylating agents, busulfan has been associated with a wide variety of specific and non-specific cutaneous changes. Diffuse hyperpigmentation has been noted (see Figure 5.4), which resolves with discontinuation of therapy. Systemic mechlorethamine (nitrogen mustard) has no cutaneous toxicity. However, when applied topically for cutaneous T-cell lymphomas, telangiectasias, hyperpigmentation and allergic contact dermatitis may occur. The development of more effective, safer alternative agents has rendered busulfan and mechlorethamine to essentially historical interest only or narrow

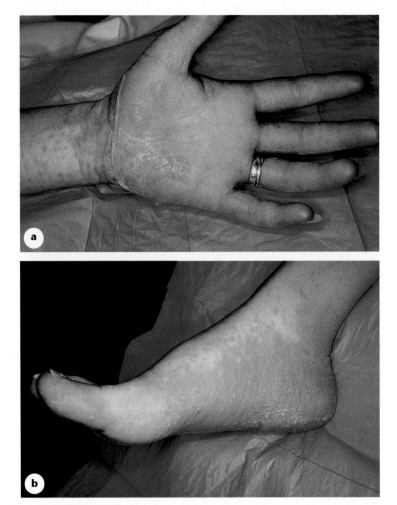

Fig. 5.4 (a,b) Dermatitis, skin rashes and hyperpigmentation: hand–foot syndrome related to 5-fluorouracil chemotherapy in metastatic colon cancer. Note the erythema, oedema, rash and early skin desquamation. Severe pain is associated with this toxic reaction.

indications (busulfan in allogeneic bone marrow transplant for haematological malignancies). Cyclophosphamide, ifosfamide and melphalan produce hyperpigmentation of nails, teeth, gingiva and skin.

The antimetabolites methotrexate and 5-FU are frequently associated with cutaneous reactions. In contrast, the purine antimetabolites

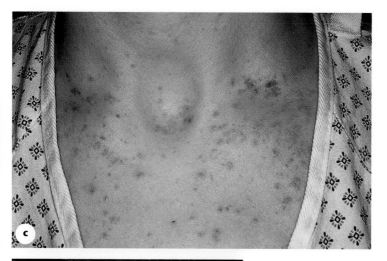

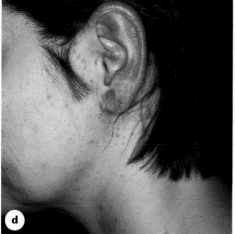

Fig. 5.4 *Continued* (c,d) Skin reaction to Ara-C. Note the erythematous macular rash on the chest and diffuse erythema and oedema of the ears in this 22-year-old woman receiving Ara-C for acute leukaemia.

6-mercaptopurine, 6-thioguanine, cladribine, fludarabine and pento-statin are devoid of cutaneous toxicity. Methotrexate, a folate antago-nist, may cause reactivation of ultraviolet burns when given in close proximity to previous sun exposure. This is not prevented by leucov-orin, a reduced folate that prevents the myelosuppression and stom-

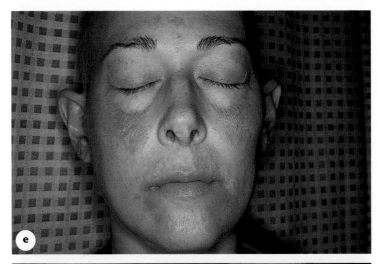

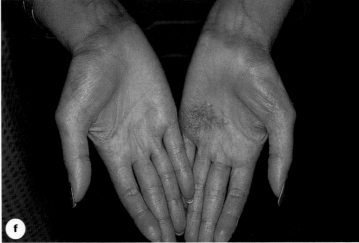

Fig. 5.4 *Continued* (e,f) Skin reaction to docetaxel. Note periorbital and malar flush along with erythema and oedema of the palms in this patient.

atitis of high doses of methotrexate. Methotrexate should be given more than a week after a significant solar burn. It may cause stomatitis and cutaneous ulcerations at high dose, despite the use of leucovorin. Extensive epidermal necrolysis may occur and be fatal. Multiple areas of vesiculation and erosion over pressure areas have been noticed.

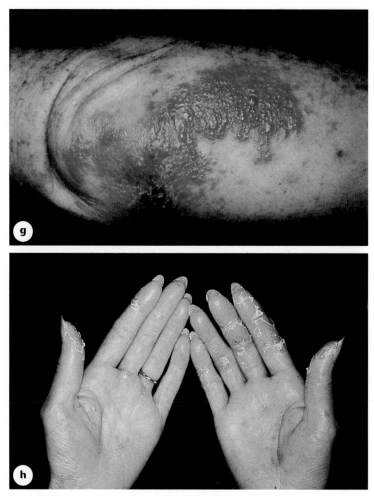

Fig. 5.4 *Continued* (**g,h**) Cutaneous reactions to bleomycin include raised, erythematous and pruritic lesions around pressure points, especially the elbows (**g**), as well as desquamation of skin (**h**).

5-FU is an antimetabolite with steric properties similar to uracil. Like methotrexate, 5-FU produces increased sensitivity to ultraviolet-induced toxic reactions in a large number of patients, over 35% in one study. Enhanced sunburn erythema and increased posterythema hyper-pigmentation characterize these reactions. A hyperpigmentation reac-tion over the veins in which the drug is administered may occur. This is

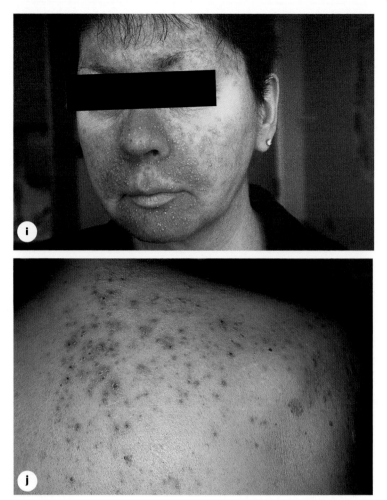

Fig. 5.4 *Continued* (i,j) Acneiform skin lesions occur in patients on gefitinib, especially on the face (i), chest and back (j). These rashes may regress when the drug is temporarily withheld or the dose is lowered. Similar skin reactions occur after actinomycin D and corticosteroids.

probably hyperpigmentation secondary to chemical phlebitis due to chemotherapeutic agents in the superficial venous system. Nail and generalized skin hyperpigmentation have been reported with 5-FU. Occasionally, acute inflammation of existing actinic keratosis is seen in patients receiving 5-FU. This differs from a drug reaction in that it occurs in discrete inflamed regions only in sun-exposed areas, not in a

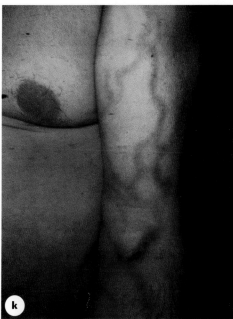

Fig. 5.4 *Continued* **(k)** Hyperpigmentation of the skin along veins occurs after the use of many chemotherapeutic agents, including Navelbine, actinomycin D and 5-fluorouracil infusion, as in this patient. In many cases, the veins become sclerotic due to thrombophlebitis. **(l–n)** Hyperpigmentation of the skin after 5-fluorouracil **(l)**, *Continued*

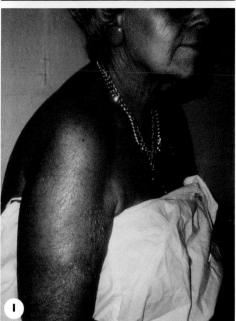

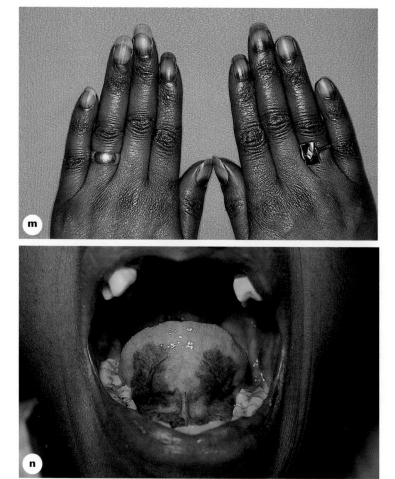

Fig. 5.4 *Continued* Hyperpigmentation of the skin occurs after adriamycin and other drugs (**m**), while increased pigment in the mucous membranes (**n**) and nails (**m**) is mainly related to adriamycin. (Also see Fig. 5.6b).

generalized distribution. The end result is usually the disappearance of the actinic keratosis as a result of an inflammatory infiltration into the atypical epidermis and resultant removal of atypical cells.

When 5-FU is given by intravenous continuous infusion, the most common dose-limiting toxicity is erythromalagia, the so-called hand–foot syndrome (see Figure 5.4). The hands and feet become red, oedematous and often painful. The skin often peels afterwards. The nails become dry and brittle and develop linear cracks. This may occur at doses less than those that produce the hand–foot syndrome. Other drugs that can result in this syndrome include new, targeted therapy drugs, such as sorafenib and sunitinib, which have multiple targets including vascular endothelial growth factor (VEGF) receptor. A similar reaction occurs with 5-FU or 5-FU prodrugs administered orally on a daily schedule. Capecitabine, an oral prodrug that is eventually converted to 5-FU intracellularly, produces erythromalagia as its most common toxicity. Interestingly, oral 5-FU does not produce this syndrome when combined with enyluracil, an irreversible inhibitor of dihydropyrimidine dehydrogenase, the major enzyme in 5-FU catabolism.

High doses of cytosine arabinoside may produce ocular toxicity through an ulcerating keratoconjunctivitis. This may be prevented by the prophylactic administration of steroid eyedrops. Excessive lacrimation may be noted with 5-FU therapy due to lacrimal duct stenosis. This is corrected by surgical dilatation of the duct.

The indirect acting anticancer drugs may produce superficial cutaneous toxicity. The anthracyclines doxorubicin, daunorubicin, epirubicin and idarubicin produce complete alopecia. Radiation recall reactions are frequent, even when the two modalities are separated by years. Skin, nail and mucous membrane hyperpigmentation may be striking; these may be localized or general. Hyperpigmentation of the hands, feet and face may occur in patients of African descent. Liposomal anthracyclines, such as Doxil (doxorubicin) and Daunosome (daunorubicin), may produce a severe erythromayalagia with palmar and plantar erythema and desquamation similar to 5-FU. Actinomycin D produces a characteristic skin eruption in many patients. Beginning 3–5 days after drug administration, patients develop facial erythema followed by papules, pustules and plugged follicles similar to the open comedones of acne. This eruption is benign, self-limited and not a reason to stop therapy. A similar acneiform skin rash occurs in patients taking the new oral epidermal growth factor receptor inhibitors such as gefitinib and erlotinib (see Figure 5.4). In most patients the rash is mild and may regress with continued treatment. When severe, the skin lesions will rapidly regress with discontinuation of the drug. Topical steroids and antibiotics may be indicated.

Bleomycin is actually a mixture of peptides isolated from *Streptomyces verticullus*. Its most common toxic effects involve the lungs and skin because of high concentrations in these organs due to the deficiency of the catabolic enzyme bleomycin hydrolase in these tissues. Cutaneous toxicity occurs in the majority of patients treated with bleomycin doses in excess of 200 mg. Bleomycin causes a morbilliform eruption 30 minutes to 3 hours after administration in approximately 10% of patients (see Figure 5.4). It most likely represents a transient hypersensitivity response (it may be accompanied by fever). Linear or "flagellate" hyperpigmentation may occur on the trunk. This may likewise represent postinflammatory hyperpigmentation. Bleomycin may cause a scleroderma-like eruption of the skin. Infiltrative plaques, nodules and linear bands of the hands have been described. Pathological findings include dermal sclerosis and appendage entrapment similar to that seen in scleroderma. These changes are reversible when the drug is stopped.

Etoposide has relatively few cutaneous manifestations at standard doses (<600 mg/m^2). At higher doses (1800–4200 mg/m^2), a generalized pruritic, erythematous, maculopapular rash occurs in approximately 25% of patients. The most severe toxicity occurs at the highest doses. In these patients, an intense, well-defined palmar erythema develops. Affected areas become oedematous, red and painful. Bullus formation and desquamation follow. The severity of the reaction is related to dose. A short course (3–5 days) of corticosteroids controls the symptoms.

Sorafenib and a related drug, sunitinib malate, are oral multi-targeted receptor tyrosine kinase inhibitors that block signal transduction through the *raf* kinases, vascular endothelial growth factor receptor 2 (VEGFR2) and the platelet-derived growth factor receptors. At the recommended dose there is a 33% incidence of skin rashes or desquamation, 27% incidence of hand–foot syndome and 22% incidence of alopecia (all grades of severity).[6]

Cutaneous rashes are the most common toxicities encountered with gefitinib and erlotinib. The chimeric monoclonal antibodies cetuximab and panitumumab are associated with dermatological toxicity. The severity and extent of the skin changes, including dry skin, desquamation, erythema, nail changes and acneiform eruptions varies from report to report and no consistent grading system for incidence and severity is universally agreed upon. There is neutrophil and macrophage infiltration of the dermis and hair follicles, with thinning of the epidermis and stratum corneum. The incidence and severity is dose-dependent. Certain epidermal growth factor receptor polymorphisms increase the incidence of developing a rash. For erlotinib, cetuximab and panitumumab, several studies support a positive correlation between development of a rash and response, and rash and survival.[7] Management is usually supportive with creams, including 1% clindamycin, 5% benzoyl peroxide and systemic antibiotics when there is evidence of infection, including tetracycline and amoxicillin/clavulinate. These should be used only when necessary.

SKIN ULCERATION AND EXTRAVASATION

Vesicant reactions from extravasated cancer chemotherapeutic agents are one of the most debilitating complications seen with cancer therapy (see Figure 5.5). The anthracyclines, especially doxorubicin, are particularly noted for an intense inflammatory chemical cellulitis caused by

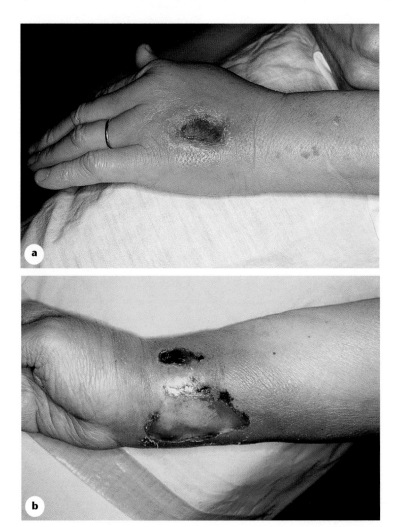

Fig. 5.5 (a–d) Extravasation of drugs and skin ulcers occurs with vesicant drugs. Acute changes with adriamycin (**a,b**)

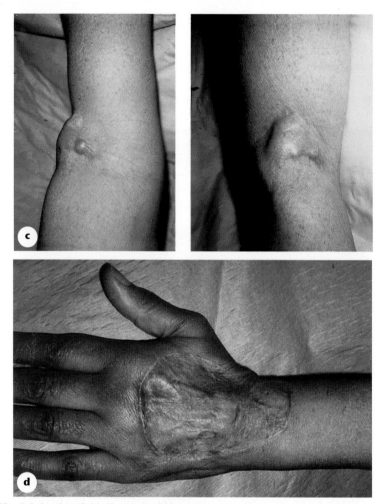

Fig. 5.5 *Continued* (c) Chronic healed scarring with adriamycin, **(d)** mitomycin-C. Other drugs include actinomycin D, vincristine and Navelbine. Immediate medical attention is necessary and sometimes skin grafts are required (see text).

subcutaneous extravasation. This results in ulceration and necrosis of affected tissue. No local measures have proven unequivocally helpful once the accident has occurred. Doxorubicin should be stopped immediately but the intravenous line left in place. Dilution of doxorubicin with sodium bicarbonate and the local installation of steroids prior to catheter withdrawal are standard measures but their efficacy is uncertain. Rest and warm compresses are recommended. If healing does not proceed well, excision of the affected area and surgical grafting are recommended to avoid excess morbidity. Other agents with vesicant properties include the vinca alkaloids (vincristine, vinblastine, vinorelbine) and actinomycin. General recommendations for the administration of vesicant drugs include the use of veins as far away from the hands and joints as possible and that the intravenous line be able to infuse at a rapid rate and have a good blood return. The use of venous access devices is accepted as appropriate in this situation unless contraindicated on specific clinical grounds.

Generalized skin ulceration is an infrequent, albeit dramatic, occurrence. Mucocutaneous ulcerations are frequently noted with bleomycin. These begin as oedema and erythema over pressure points such as the elbows, knees and fingertips and in intertrigenous areas such as the groin and axillae. These areas then proceed to shallow ulcerations. These ulcerations may also occur in the oral cavity. Biopsy shows epidermal degeneration and necrosis with dermal oedema. Total epidermal necrosis can even be found without any dermal changes. This suggests that the epidermal toxicity is the primary event.

NAIL CHANGES

Banding of the nails is the appearance of linear horizontal depressions in the nails that occur as a result of growth interruptions in the nail germinal cell layer by a cytostatic effect from the administration of cancer chemotherapy agents. These occur in other disease settings and are called Beau's lines (see Figure 5.6). The direct-acting alkylating agents cyclophosphamide, ifosfamide and melphalan may also produce hyperpigmentation of nails. The nails may exhibit linear or transverse banding or hyperpigmentation. These changes begin proximally and progress distally and clear, proximally to distally, when the agents are discontinued. Similar effects are seen with the indirect–acting anthracyclines, such as doxorubicin, and bleomycin. The anthracyclines may cause hyperpigmentation of the hyponychia (the soft layer of skin beneath the nail), especially in dark-skinned persons.

Onycholysis is separation of the nail plate from the nail bed (see Figure 5.6). Anthracyclines, anthracenediones and taxanes are the drugs most frequently associated with onycholysis. The combination of these agents is most frequently reported with onycholysis. Most of the reports are associated with docetaxel, either administered weekly or every 3

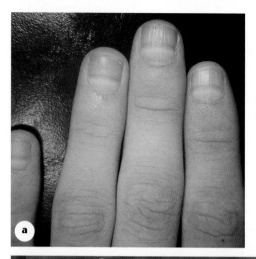

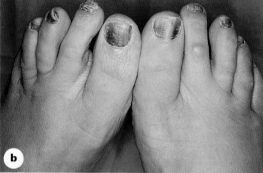

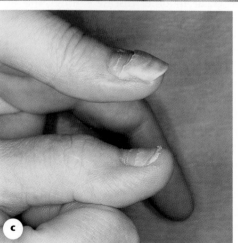

Fig. 5.6 Nail changes are often seen after prolonged chemotherapy. (**a**) Banding of the nails results from growth interruptions in the nail germinal cell layer by the cytostatic effect of chemotherapy. These white bands (called Mee's lines) will grow outward eventually. Beau's lines are transverse grooves across the nail plate due to temporary nail matrix malfunction, seen with chemotherapy or associated with other illnesses (acute coronary or severe febrile episodes). Nail hyperpigmentation occurs occasionally after prolonged use of adriamycin (**b**) especially in people with dark skin. Onycholysis or separation of the nail from its bed is associated with use of adriamycin (**c**), cyclophosphamide and the taxanes.

weeks. These changes occur after hyperpigmentation of the hyponychia, often with hyperkeratosis and splinter haemorrhages. Ultraviolet light may be a facilitating factor. Onycholysis can occur within weeks or months of the initiation of therapy.

RADIATION RECALL

Radiation recall dermatitis is a cutaneous toxicity that develops in patients with prior exposure to therapeutic doses of radiation and subsequent treatment with a cancer chemotherapeutic agent (see Figure 5.7). These reactions occur in the previously irradiated field and not elsewhere. A previous cutaneous reaction at the time of irradiation is not a prerequisite. The onset of symptoms is days to weeks after drug treatment and can occur any time after radiation, even years later. Cutaneous manifestations include erythema with maculopapular eruptions, vesiculation and desquamation. The intensity of the cutaneous response can vary from a mild rash to skin necrosis. Radiation recall reactions in other organs can produce gastrointestinal mucosal inflammation (stomatitis, oesophagitis, enteritis, proctitis), pneumonitis and myocarditis.

An extensive number of anticancer agents have been implicated in radiation recall reactions. The anthracyclines (doxorubicin as an example), bleomycin, dactinomycin, etoposide, the taxanes, vinca alkaloids and antimetabolites (hydroxycarbamide, fluorouracil, methotrexate, gemcitabine) are the most commonly implicated in cutaneous toxicity. In addition, these skin reactions have been seen in association with targeted therapy with drugs such as gefitinib.

Methotrexate and dactinomycin are reported to cause radiation enhancement in the central nervous system (CNS). The antimetabolites doxorubicin, dactinomycin and bleomycin enhance gastrointestinal toxicity from radiation. Cyclophosphamide, taxanes, hydroxycarbamide, doxorubicin, dactinomycin, gemcitabine, cytosine arabinoside and, most importantly, bleomycin exacerbate pulmonary radiation toxicity. Optic toxicity is increased by treatment with fluorouracil and cytosine arabinoside. Radiation lowers the dose of doxorubicin that produces cardiomyopathy.

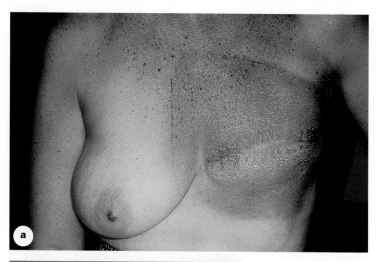

Fig. 5.7 Radiation recall dermatitis may occur in a radiotherapy treatment field after systemic chemotherapy, with development of hyperaemia and then hyperpigmentation in the healing phase (**a**). The patient in (**a**) received adjuvant Alkeran (melphalan) 1 month after postoperative radiation to the chest wall. (**b**) This patient had radiation therapy to the lower spine for bone metastases from breast cancer and developed recall dermatitis 6 months later, when gemcitabine was administered.

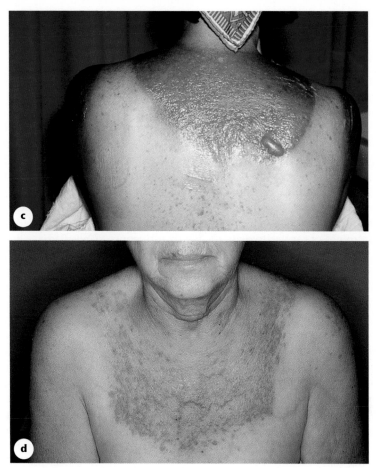

Fig. 5.7 *Continued* (**c**) Chemotherapy can also sensitize the skin to adverse reactions to solar radiation. This young woman developed severe dermatitis in a sun-exposed area while taking methotrexate. (**d**) This patient also developed acute dermatitis in a sun-exposed area while receiving 5-fluorouracil.

ORGAN TOXICITY

CARDIAC AND CARDIOVASCULAR TOXICITY

Cardiotoxicity is a well-recognized consequence of anthracycline use, especially doxorubicin because of its wide spectrum of antineoplastic therapy. This peculiar and potentially lethal problem can be classified as acute or chronic. The acute toxicity is usually asymptomatic arrhythmias, including heart block. Acute myopericarditis occurs at low total doses in an idiosyncratic fashion or at high single doses >110–120 mg/m^2. Fever, pericarditis and congestive heart failure (CHF) are the clinical manifestations. Chronic cardiomyopathy is characterized by progressive myofibrillar damage with each dose, dilatation of sarcoplasmic reticulum, loss of myofibrils and myocardial necrosis/fibrosis. Various syndromes of cardiac toxicity related to antineoplastic agents have been recently reviewed in detail.[8] Imatinib mesylate used commonly in chronic myelogenous leukaemia and gastrointestinal stromal tumours, has been associated with a low incidence of cardiomyopathy syndrome.[9]

A doxorubicin total dose <550 mg/m^2 has a 1–10% occurrence of CHF (daunorubicin 900–1000 mg/m^2), a 40% incidence at 800 mg/m^2 of doxorubicin, and the incidence of CHF approaches 100% at 1 g/m^2. Cardiac function is tested using non-invasive techniques to measure the resting and exercise ejection fraction, including radionuclide ventriculograms and echocardiograms, or invasively by cardiac biopsy. Factors that increase the risk of developing CHF include pre-existing heart disease, hypertension and cardiac radiation therapy. Concomitant dosing with trastuzamab increases the cardiac toxicity of doxorubicin. Cardiac toxicity is a function of *peak* dose level, so continuous infusions or weekly dosing decrease the risk. Desrazoxane, an iron chelator, decreases cardiotoxicity and is approved for use.

Biochemical mechanisms implicated include calcium-mediated damage to the sarcoplasmic reticulum which increases calcium ion (Ca^{++}) release with increased Ca^{++} uptake in mitochondria in preference to ATP. Lipid peroxidations of the sarcoplasmic reticulum, which decrease high Ca^{++} binding sites, and lipid peroxidation due to drug $^\bullet$Fe^{3+} complexes with hydroxyl (OH) radical generation may contribute to cardiotoxicity. The heart has no catalase, and anthracyclines decrease glutathione peroxidase activity, which increases the sensitivity of the myocardium to oxidative damage.

Idarubicin and epirubicin have less cardiotoxicity but are still capable of causing cardiotoxicity. High-dose cyclophosphamide, at doses

>60 mg/kg as used in bone marrow transplantation, can cause a haemor-rhagic cardiomyopathy. Paclitaxel produces clinically insignificant atrial arrhythmias. Agents that can produce arterial smooth muscle spasm may produce ischaemic myocardial infarction in the absence of fixed coronary vascular disease. These agents include 5-FU, vincristine and vinblastine.

Combination chemotherapy in colorectal cancer with bevacizumab has been associated with an incidence (1–3%) of ischaemic cardiac events above that observed with conventional therapy alone. This increase in cardiovascular events, while of low overall incidence, nonetheless represents about a 3-fold increase.[10]

Sunitinib has a 10% incidence of usually reversible cardiomyopathy. Patients can often be treated with lower doses if and when symptoms resolve.[11]

Hypertension has been recognized as a class effect for agents that target VEGFR2. Hypertension is so common that it serves as a pharmacodynam-ic endpoint in the early development of agents of this class. Hypertension of a moderate degree (grade 2, recurrent or persistent, symptomatic increase of diastolic blood pressure >200 mmHg or to >150/100 mmHg or requiring monotherapy) or severe degree (grade 3, requiring more than one agent or more intensive therapy) occurs in 10–25% of patients receiv-ing bevacizumab, sorafenib or sunitinib. Patients with pre-existing or bor-derline hypertension are more susceptible. No specific treatment algo-rithmn has yet been applied to the management of these patients.

PULMONARY TOXICITY

Bleomycin produces pulmonary toxicity, which is the major problem with subacute or chronic interstitial pneumonitis complicated by late-stage fibrosis (see Figure 5.8). The incidence is 3–5% with doses <450 u/m^2, in patients over 70, with emphysema and after high single doses (>25 u/m^2). The incidence rises to 10% at doses >450 mg/m^2, but can occur at cumu-lative doses <100 mg. Pulmonary injury can occur during high FiO_2 and volume overload during surgery for many years after exposure.

Toxicity results from free radicals produced by an intercalated Fe(II)–bleomycin–O_2 complex between DNA strands. Intercalation of drug into the DNA is the first step; then Fe(II) is oxidized and O_2 is reduced to oxygen ($^{\bullet}O_2{}_-$) or hydroxyl radicals $^{\bullet}$OH. DNA cleavage occurs after the acti-vated bleomycin complex is assembled. Strand breakage absolutely requires O_2, which is converted to $O_2{}_-$ and $^{\bullet}$OH, and peroxidation prod-ucts of DNA (and protein) are formed. Free radical scavengers and super-oxide dismutase inhibit DNA breakage. Bleomycin is hydrolyzed by

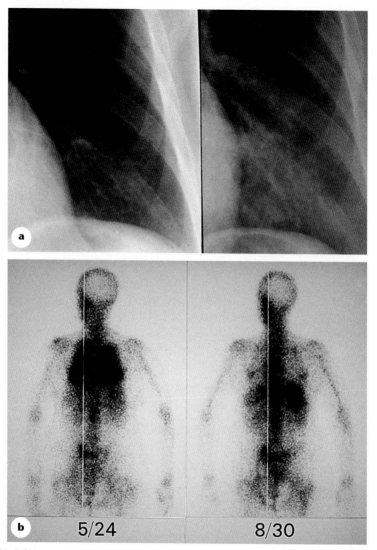

Fig. 5.8 Organ toxicity. Non-mucocutaneous toxicity of chemotherapeutic agents is covered in the text. The lung may be affected by several agents including bleomycin. (a) The earliest radiographic changes are linear infiltrates in the lower lung fields. (b) Gallium-67 uptake is quite striking but is reversible, as this serial study demonstrates.

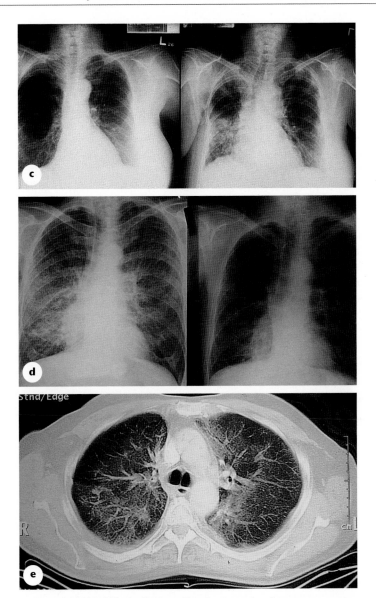

Fig. 5.8 *Continued* (c) While usually dose related, progressive changes may occur resulting in fibrosis and pulmonary insufficiency. Other drugs such as alkylating agents and high-dose methotrexate may result in diffuse infiltrates (d), which were reversible 4 months later. (e) In this patient several courses of gemcitabine resulted in acute dyspnoea and decreased oxygen saturation. Evaluation with lung biopsy and other studies showed no evidence of infection, pulmonary emboli or other diagnosable disease. Use of prednisone led to rapid improvement and regression of the interstitial infiltrates.

bleomycin hydrolase, a cysteine present in normal and malignant cells but decreased in lung and skin.

Busulfan, mitomycin C and carmustine are direct-acting alkylating agents that can cause chronic interstitial pneumonitis and fibrosing alveolitis. This chronic fibrosis produces the clinical picture of progressive, often fatal, restrictive lung disease. The symptoms occur insidiously, often after prolonged therapy. The chronic use of busulfan for the treatment of chronic myelogenous leukaemia is now a historical footnote but carmustine remains the mainstay of treatment for glioblastoma and anaplastic astrocytomas. Cyclophosphamide has been implicated in chronic pulmonary toxicity but rarely as a single agent, more often after radiation.

The antimetabolite methotrexate may produce an acute eosinophilic pneumonitis, which represents an allergic reaction. Cytosine arabinoside and gemcitabine (2',2'-difluoro-2'-deoxycytidine) may also cause an acute pneumonitis, which may be fatal if unrecognized. In these circumstances, withdrawal of the offending agent, supportive care and corticosteroids may prevent a fatal outcome.[12] Some of the reported pulmonary syndromes associated with chemotherapy drugs are noted in Table 5.1.

Table 5.1 Pulmonary syndromes associated with specific cancer chemotherapy drugs

Syndrome	Associated cancer chemotherapy drugs
Pulmonary capillary leak	Interleukin-2, recombinant tumour necrosis factor alpha, cytarabine, mitomycin
Asthma	Interleukin-2, vinca alkaloids plus mitomycin
Bronchiolitis obliterans organizing pneumonia	Bleomycin, cyclophosphamide, methotrexate, mitomycin
Hypersensitivity pneumonitis	Busulfan, bleomycin, etoposide, methotrexate, mitomycin, procarbazine
Interstitial pneumonia/fibrosis	Bleomycin, busulfan, chlorambucil, cyclophosphamide, melphalan, methotrexate, nitrosureas, procarbazine, vinca alkaloids (with mitomycin), gefitinib, erlotinib
Pleural effusion	Bleomycin, busulfan, interleukin-2, methotrexate, mitomycin, procarbazine
Pulmonary vascular injury	Busulfan, nitrosureas

Adapted with permission from Belknap SM, Kuzel TM, Yarnold PR, et al: Clinical features and correlates of gemcitabine-associated lung injury. Cancer 2006; 106: 2051–2057

Both erlotinib and gefitinib, new oral agents targeted at the epidermal growth factor receptor 1, both have a low (<1%) but real incidence of interstitial pneumonitis that resolves if the agent is stopped. The highest incidence is in Asian patients, where 3.5% of patients may develop interstitial disease also referred to as ground glass opacities, which carries a mortalilty of 1.6%.[13]

HEPATOTOXICITY

The liver is a frequent organ for toxicity with cancer chemotherapeutic agents. Centrilobular hepatocyte injury is the frequent histological finding, elevated transaminases the biochemical manifestation. Antimetabolite drugs such as cytosine arabinoside, methotrexate, hydroxycarbamide and 6-Mercaptopurine are all associated with hepatic injury. 6-Mercaptopurine produces a cholestatic picture, with an elevated alkaline phosphatase and bilirubin. L-Asparaginase and carmustine cause hepatotoxicity as well. The injury reverses with discontinuation of the drug. Chronic methotrexate administration, such as in the treatment of autoimmune diseases, is associated with irreversible fibrosis and cirrhosis.

Hepatic vascular injury is another type of injury to the liver associated with cancer chemotherapeutic agents. Hepatic veno-occlusive disease may occur in up to 20% of patients receiving high-dose chemotherapy in conjunction with bone marrow transplantation, with a mortality up to 50%. Jaundice, ascites and hepatomegaly are the full manifestations of veno-occlusive disease but right upper quadrant pain and weight gain occur more frequently. Obliteration of the central hepatic venules and resulting pressure necrosis of the hepatocytes is seen at autopsy. Many regimens and many individual drugs have been implicated. With busulfan, adjustment of the plasma concentration–time profile may reduce the risk. Dacarbazine, a monofunctional alkylating agent, may produce an eosinophilic centrilobular injury with hepatic vein thromboses.

GASTROINTESTINAL TOXICITY

Chemotherapy-induced diarrhoea has been described with several drugs including the fluoropyrimidines (particularly 5-FU), irinotecan, methotrexate and cisplatin. However, it is the major toxicity of regimens containing a fluoropyrimidine and/or irinotecan that can be dose limiting. Both 5-FU and irinotecan cause acute damage to the intestinal mucosa, leading to loss of epithelium. 5-FU causes a mitotic arrest of crypt cells, leading to an increase in the ratio of immature secretory crypt cells to mature villous enterocytes. The increased volume of fluid that leaves the small bowel exceeds the absorptive capacity of the colon, leading to clinically significant diarrhoea.

In patients treated with irinotecan, early-onset diarrhoea, which occurs during or within several hours of drug infusion in 45–50% of patients, is cholinergically mediated. This effect is thought to be due to structural similarity with acetylcholine. In contrast, late irinotecan-associated diarrhoea is not cholinergically mediated. The pathophysiology of late diarrhoea appears to be multifactorial with contributions from dysmotility and secretory factors as well as a direct toxic effect of the drug on the intestinal mucosa.

Irinotecan produces mucosal changes associated with apoptosis, such as epithelial vacuolization, and goblet cell hyperplasia, suggestive of mucin hypersecretion. These changes appear to be related to the accumulation of the active metabolite of irinotecan, SN-38, in the intestinal mucosa. SN-38 is glucuronidated in the liver and is then excreted in the bile. The conjugated metabolite SN-38G does not appear to cause diarrhoea. However, SN-38G can be deconjugated in the intestines by β-glucuronidase present in intestinal bacteria. A direct correlation has been noted between mucosal damage and either low glucuronidation rates or increased intestinal β-glucuronidase activity. Severe toxicity has been described following irinotecan therapy in patients with Gilbert's syndrome, who have defective hepatic glucuronidation. Experimental studies have shown that inhibition of intestinal β-glucuronidase activity with antibiotics protects against mucosal injury and ameliorates the diarrhoea.

Several recently approved receptor tyrosine kinase inhibitors have diarrhoea associated with use, including sorafenib, sunitinib, erlotinib and gefitinib. The frequency varies from 30–40% with less than 5% grade 3 (severe).[14] Also, rare cases of gastrointestinal perforation have been reported using new agents with several mechanisms of action, including inhibitors of tumour vasculature.[15] Hypertension and rare strokes are also side effects that have been reported.

NEUROTOXICITY

Neurotoxicity from cancer chemotherapeutic agents is an increasingly recognized consequence of cancer treatment. The toxicities observed may affect the brain and spinal cord (CNS), peripheral nerves or the supporting neurological tissues such as the meninges. Neurotoxicity from cancer therapeutic drugs must be distinguished from the effects of space-occupying metastatic lesions, toxic metabolic effects from disorders of blood chemistry, adjunctive drugs (such as opiate narcotics) and paraneoplastic syndromes. Toxicity may be acute, subacute or chronic, reversible or irreversible.

The direct-acting alkylating agents ifosfamide and carmustine cause somnolence, confusion and coma at high doses. The toxicity of ifosfamide is secondary to accumulation of a metabolite, chlorethyl aldehyde, in cerebrospinal fluid. Renal dysfunction may cause CNS toxicity at low doses when acidosis results in increased chlorethyl aldehyde levels.

Damage from the antimetabolite methotrexate occurs in three forms and is worse when given intrathecally with radiation. Chemical arachnoiditis, characterized by headache, fever and nuchal rigidity, is the most common and most acute toxicity. This may be due to additives in the diluent (benzoic acid in sterile water). Subacute toxicity is delayed for 2–3 weeks after administration and is characterized by extremity motor paralysis, cranial nerve palsy seizures and coma. This is due to prolonged exposure to high doses of methotrexate. Chronic demyelinating encephalitis produces dementia and spasticity. There is cortical thinning with enlarged ventricles and cerebral calcifications. Types 2 and 3 may be increased after irradiation especially if concomitant systemic therapy with high (or intermediate) doses is used.

Cytosine arabinoside, when given at high doses, produces cerebral and cerebellar dysfunction due to Purkinje cell necrosis and damage. At standard doses, leukoencephalopathy occurs rarely. When given intrathecally, cytosine arabinoside can produce transverse myelitis with resulting paralysis. 5-FU may produce acute cerebellar toxicity due to inhibition of aconintase, an enzyme in the cerebellar Krebs cycle. The purine adenine deaminase inhibitors pentostatin and fludarabine may produce several types of neurotoxicity. Pentostatin produces somnolence and coma at high doses. Fludarabine may cause delayed-onset coma or cortical blindness at high doses, peripheral neuropathy at low doses. Peripheral neuropathy is a frequent toxicity encountered with many cancer chemotherapeutic agents of many classes. Cisplatin and oxaliplatin, the vinca alkaloids and the taxanes all produce peripheral neuropathy in a cumulative dose-dependent manner (see p.73-76 for more on oxaliplatin-related neurotoxicity).

NEPHROTOXICITY

One of the most serious side-effects of chemotherapeutic agents is nephrotoxicity. Any part of the kidney structure (e.g. the glomerulus, the tubules, the interstitium or the renal microvasculature) could be vulnerable to damage. The clinical manifestations of nephrotoxicity can range from an asymptomatic elevation of serum creatinine to acute renal failure requiring dialysis. Intravascular volume depletion secondary to ascites, oedema or external losses, concomitant use of nephrotoxic drugs, urinary tract obstruction secondary to the underlying malignancy, tumour infiltration of the kidney and intrinsic renal disease can potentiate renal dysfunction in the cancer patient.

Platinum compounds are the agents most associated with renal toxicity. Cisplatin is one of the most commonly used and effective chemotherapeutic agents available and also the best studied antineoplastic nephrotoxic drug. It is a potent tubular toxin, particularly in a low chloride environment, such as the interior of cells. Cell death results via apoptosis or necrosis as DNA-damaged cells enter the cell cycle. Approximately 25–35% of patients will develop a mild and partially reversible decline in renal function after the first course of therapy. The incidence and severity of renal failure increase with subsequent courses, eventually becoming in part irreversible. As a result, discontinuing therapy is generally indicated in those patients who develop a progressive rise in plasma creatinine concentration. In addition to this rise, potentially irreversible hypomagnesaemia due to urinary magnesium wasting may occur in over one-half of cases.

There is suggestive evidence that the nephrotoxicity of cisplatin can be diminished by vigorous hydration and perhaps by giving the drug in a hypertonic solution. A high chloride concentration may minimize both the formation of the highly reactive platinum compounds described above and the uptake of cisplatin by the renal tubular cells. Amifostine, an organic thiophosphate, appears to diminish cisplatin-induced toxicity by donating a protective thiol group, an effect that is highly selective for normal, but not malignant, tissue. Discontinuation of platinum therapy once the plasma creatinine concentration begins to rise should prevent progressive renal failure.

Carboplatin has been synthesized as a non-nephrotoxic platinum analogue, but even though it is less nephrotoxic, it is not free of potential for renal injury. Hypomagnesaemia appears to be the most common manifestation of nephrotoxicity. Other, less common renal side-effects include recurrent salt wasting. No significant clinical nephrotoxicity due to oxaliplatin has yet been reported. Limited data have shown no exacerbation of pre-existing mild renal impairment. Studies of oxaliplatin in patients with progressive degrees of renal failure are in progress.

Cyclophosphamide may produce significant side-effects involving the urinary bladder (haemorrhagic cystitis). The primary renal effect of this agent is hyponatraemia, which is due to impairment of the ability of the kidney to excrete water. The mechanism appears to be due to a direct effect of cyclophosphamide on the distal tubule and not to increased levels of antidiuretic hormone. Hyponatraemia usually occurs acutely and resolves upon discontinuation of the drug (approximately 24 hours). It is recommended that isotonic saline be infused prior to cyclophosphamide administration in order to ameliorate this effect.

Ifosfamide nephrotoxicity has a primary renal effect to produce tubular renal toxicity. The damage produced by ifosfamide is concentrated in the proximal renal tubule and a Fanconi syndrome has been observed after therapy. Other clinical syndromes that have been associated with ifosfamide include nephrogenic diabetes insipidus, renal tubular acidosis and rickets. Pre-existing renal disease is an important risk factor for ifosfamide nephrotoxicity.

Carmustine, lomustine and semustine are lipid-soluble nitrosureas, which have been used against brain tumours. The exact mechanism of nephrotoxicity, however, is incompletely understood. High doses of semustine in children and adults have been associated with progressive renal dysfunction to marked renal insufficiency 3–5 years after therapy. The characteristic histological changes include glomerular sclerosis without immune deposits and interstitial fibrosis. The incidence of nephrotoxicity was reported at 26% in patients with malignant melanoma treated with methyl CCNU in the adjuvant setting. Nephrotoxicity has been reported in 65–75% of patients treated with streptozotocin for prolonged periods of time. Proteinuria is often the first sign of renal damage. This is followed by signs of proximal tubular damage, such as phosphaturia, glycosuria, aminoaciduria, uricosuria and bicarbonaturia. Renal toxicity lasts approximately 2–3 weeks after discontinuing the drug.

The most common form of nephrotoxicity associated with mitomycin C is haemolytic uraemic syndrome. It has been reported in patients who were treated with total doses of mitomycin C in excess of 60 mg/m^2. The renal damage caused by this antineoplastic agent appears to be direct endothelial damage. The incidence of this syndrome ranges from 4% to 6% of patients who receive this drug alone or in combination.

Low or standard doses of methotrexate are usually not associated with renal toxicity, unless patients have underlying renal dysfunction. High doses (1–15 g/m^2) are associated with a 47% incidence of renal toxicity, accompanied by methotrexate crystals in the urine. The mechanism for methotrexate-induced nephrotoxicity is explained in part by its limited solubility at an acid pH, which leads to intratubular precipitation. Patients who are volume depleted and excrete an acidic urine are at higher risk for nephrotoxicity. With aggressive hydration and urine alkalinization, the incidence of renal failure with high doses of methotrexate can be decreased. The clinical picture of methotrexate-induced renal failure is that of a non-oliguric renal failure. Preventive measures when using high doses of methotrexate include aggressive intravenous hydration with saline and urine alkalinization with sodium bicarbonate to maintain a urine pH around 7.0. If renal failure develops, methotrexate levels will increase and the risk of systemic toxicity will also be enhanced. In addition to supportive measures, patients should be started on folinic acid rescue, until levels of methotrexate fall below 0.5 uM.

VEGF or VEGFR2-targeted agents produce albuminuria in 10–25% of patients, sometimes to nephrotic range. The exact mechanism has not been elucidated but studies in mice with conditional expression of VEGF in the podocytes confirms a major role for VEGF in endothelial development and maintainence of a fenestrated endothelium.[16] Like hypertension, this appears to be a class effect but the factors associated with occurrence and severity are unknown. If clinically significant, decreasing the dose or discontinuation of drug are the only current approaches.

LATE COMPLICATIONS OF CANCER CHEMOTHERAPY

As cancer therapy has become increasingly effective and more patients live longer, late complications have become apparent separate from the direct toxic effects on organ system function described above. Gonadal dysfunction is one. In males, the primary lesion is depletion of germinal epithelium of seminiferous tubules with marked decrease in testicular volume, oligo- or azoospermia and infertility. There is an increase in follicle-stimulating hormone (FSH) and occasionally in luteinizing hormone (LH). No change is seen in serum testosterone. Alkylating agents (and irradiation) are the most damaging and toxicity is dose related. About 80% of males with Hodgkin's disease treated with MOPP are oligo-azoospermic. About half recover in up to 4 years. Procarbazine is a major offender. Anthracyclines also cause azoospermia in a dose-related fashion. In females, the primary lesion is ovarian fibrosis and follicle destruction. Amenorrhoea ensues, with increase in FSH and LH and a decrease in oestradiol leading to vaginal atrophy and endometrial hypoplasia. Onset and duration are dose and age related. Alkylating agents (and irradiation) again are the worst offenders.

In children, the prepubertal effects may be less profound and reversible in males, though the pubertal effects may be more severe with often irreversible azoospermia, decreased testosterone and increased FSH and LH. Less is known about females, but young girls appear quite resistant to alkylating agents.

No more tragic toxicity is seen with cancer chemotherapeutic agents than the induction of a second, treatment-related cancer in a patient cured of one cancer.[17,18] Of the wide variety of environmental and chemical agents causing cancer, there is one common thread in their mode of action – interaction with DNA. Clinical studies detailing this consequence of therapy have many problems, including the inherent bias of reporting index cases, the retrospective nature of many reports, the lack of reliable information on drug dosage, total amount of drug given and duration of therapy and the underlying incidence of second malignancy. The direct-acting alkylating agents are most often implicated and chronic, low-dose administration is a greater risk factor. Acute non-lymphocytic leukaemia or myelodysplasia is the best described. The indirect-acting topoisomerase II agents produce a specific 11q23 translocation.

Osteonecrosis of the jaw has been seen with increasing frequency during the past few years, related in part to chronic use of intravenous bisphophonates for advanced cancer. The incidence has been estimated at 1–10% of patients receiving these medications.[19] The pathogenesis and optimal management for osteonecrosis of the jaw are poorly understood, with multiple risk factors and various treatments involved.[20]

REFERENCES

1. Weiss RB: Toxicity of chemotherapy – the last decade. Semin Oncol 2006; 33: 1.
2. Crawford J, Cella D, Sonis ST: Managing chemotherapy-related side effects: trends in the use of cytokines and other growth factors. Oncology 2006; 20: Suppl.
3. Zorzou MP, Efstathiou E, Galani E, et al: Carboplatin hypersensitivity reactions. J Chemother 2005; 17(1): 104–110.
4. Cristaaudo A, Sera F, Severino V, et al: Occupational hypersensitivity to metal salts, including platinum, in the secondary industry. Allergy 2005; 60(2): 138–139.
5. Szebeni J: Complement activation-related pseudoallergy: a new class of drug induced acute immune toxicity. Toxicology 2005; 216: 106–121.
6. Escudier B, Szczylik C, Eisen T, et al: Randomized phase III trial of the Raf kinase and VEGFR inhibitor sorafenib (BAY 43-9006) in patients with advanced renal cell carcinoma (RCC). J Clin Oncol 2005; 23(18 Suppl): abstract 4510.
7. Perez-Solar R, Saltz L. Cutaneous adverse effects with HER1/EGFR-targeted agents: is there a silver lining? J Clin Oncol 2005; 23(24): 5235–5246.
8. Floyd JD, Nguyen DT, Lobins RL, et al: Cardiotoxicity of cancer therapy. J Clin Oncol 2005; 23: 7685–7696.

9. Kerkela R, Grazette L, Yacobi R, et al: Cardiotoxicity of the cancer therapeutic agent imatinib mesylate. Nat Med 2006; 12(8): 908–916.

10. Hurwitz H: Integrating the anti-VEGF – A humanized monoclonal antibody bevacizumab with chemotherapy in advanced colorectal cancer. Clin Colorectal Cancer 2004; 4 Suppl 2: S62–S68.

11. Motzer RJ, Hutson TE, Tomczak P, et al: Phase III randomized trial of sunitinib malate (SU11248) versus interferon alfa as first line systemic therapy for patients with metastatic renal cell carcinoma. J Clin Oncol 2006; 24 (18 Suppl): 930s abstract LBA3.

12. Belknap SM, Kuzel TM, Yarnold PR, et al: Clinical features and correlates of gemcitabine-associated lung injury. Cancer 2006; 106: 2051–2057.

13. Ando M, Okamoto I, Yamamoto N, et al: Predictive factors for interstitial lung disease, antitumor response, and survival in non-small-cell lung cancer patients treated with gefitinib. J Clin Oncol 2006; 24: 2549–2556.

14. Niho S, Kubota K, Goto K, et al: First-line single agent treatment with gefitinib in patients with advanced non-small cell lung cancer: a phase II study. J Clin Oncol 2006; 24(1): 64–69.

15. Ratain MJ, Eisen T, Stadler WM, et al: Phase II placebo-controlled randomized discontinuation trial of sorafenib in patients with metastatic renal cell carcinoma. J Clin Oncol 2006; 24: 2505–2512.

16. Erimina V, Quaggin SE: The role of VEGF-A in glomerular development and function. Curr Opin Nephrol Hypertens 2004; 13: 9–15.

17. Bhatia S, Landier W: Evaluating survivors of pediatric cancer. Cancer J 2005; 11: 340–354.

18. Hudson MM, Mertens AC, Yasui Y, et al: Health status in adults treated for childhood cancer: a report from the childhood survivor study. Am J Oncol Rev 2004; 3: 165–170.

19. Badros A, Weikel D, Salama A, et al: Osteonecrosis of the jaw in multiple myeloma patients: clinical features and risk factors. J Clin Oncol 2006; 24: 945–952.

20. Ruggiero S, Gralow J, Marx RE, et al. Practical guidelines for the prevention, diagnosis and treatment of osteonecrosis of the jaw in patients with cancer. J Oncol Pract 2006; 2: 7–14.

FURTHER READING

Adrian RM, Hood, AF, Skarin AT. Mucocutaneous reactions to antineoplastic agents. CA Cancer J Clin 1980; 30: 143–157.

Attar EC, Ervin T, Janicek M, Deykin A, Godleski J: Acute interstitial pneumonitis related to gemcitabine. J Clin Oncol 2000; 18: 697–698.

Burstein H: Radiation recall dermatitis from gemcitabine. J Clin Oncol 2000; 18: 693–694.

Chabner BA, Longo DL: Cancer Chemotherapy and Biotherapy, 2nd edn. Lippincott–Raven, Philadelphia, 1996.

Darnell J, Lodish H, Baltimore D: Molecular Cell Biology, 3rd edn. W.H. Freeman, New York, 1995.

DeVita VT, Jr, Hellman S, Rosenberg SA: Cancer: Principles and Practice of Oncology, 4th edn. Lippincott, Philadelphia, 1993.

Eder JP: Neoplasms. In: Page CP, Curtis MJ, Sutter MC, Walker MJA, Hoffman BB, eds: Integrated Pharmacology. Mosby–Times Mirror International, London, 1997: 501–522.

Hussain S, Anderson DN, Salvatti ME, et al: Onycholysis as a complication of systemic chemotherapy. Cancer 2000; 88: 2367–2371.

Perry MD: The Chemotherapy Source Book. Williams and Wilkins, Baltimore, 1992.

Skeel RT: Handbook of Cancer Chemotherapy. Little, Brown, Boston, 1991.

Sonis ST, Fey EG: Oral complications of cancer therapy. Oncology 2002; 16: 680–691.

Index